T0251648

Social Work in Ambulatory Care: New Implications for Health and Social Services

Social Work
in Ambulatory Care:
New Implications
for Health
and Social Services

Gary Rosenberg, PhD
Andrew Weissman, DSW
Editors

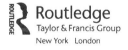

Routledge
Taylor & Francis Group
New York   London

Social Work in Ambulatory Care: New Implications for Health and Social Services has also been published as *Social Work in Health Care*, Volume 20, Number 1 1994.

First published by
The Haworth Press, Inc., 10 Alice Street, Binghamton, NY 13904-1580 USA

This edition published 2013 by Routledge
711 Third Avenue, New York, NY 10017
2 Park Square, Milton Park, Abingdon, Oxon OX14 4RN

Routledge is an imprint of the Taylor & Francis Group, an informa business

Library of Congress Cataloging-in-Publication Data

Social work in ambulatory care : new implications for health and social services / Gary Rosenberg, Andrew Weissman, editors
     p. cm.
     Papers presented at the Sixth Doris Siegel Memorial Colloquium, April 2, 1992.
     This text "has also been published as Social Work in Health Care, Volume 20, Number 1, 1994"–CIP t.p. verso.
     Includes bibliographical references and index.
     ISBN 1-56024-697-9 (acid free paper)
     1. Medical social work–United States–Congresses. 2. Ambulatory medical care–United States–Congresses. 3. Social service–United States–Congresses. I. Rosenberg, Gary. II. Weissman, Andrew, 1941– . III. Doris Siegel Memorial Colloquium (6th : 1992 : Mount Sinai Medical Center)
HV687.5.U5A75 1994
362.1'0425–dc20   94-29502
                                                           CIP

Social Work in Ambulatory Care: New Implications for Health and Social Services

CONTENTS

ABOUT THE EDITORS

Gary Rosenberg, PhD, is the Edith J. Baerwald Professor of Community Medicine (Social Work) and Senior Vice President at The Mount Sinai Medical Center, New York City. He is past President of the Society for Social Work Administrators in Health Care. Dr. Rosenberg has been elected to the Hunter College Hall of Fame and has received the Distinguished Alumni Award from Adelphi University and the Founders Day Award from New York University. In addition, he is a Fellow in the Brookdale Center on Aging, a Fellow in the New York Academy of Medicine, and a recipient of the Ida M. Cannon Award of the Society for Hospital Social Work Directors.

Andrew Weissman, DSW, is Assistant Professor in the Department of Community Medicine (Social Work) and an Administrator in the Office of the Senior Vice President at The Mount Sinai Medical Center, New York City. He is a past Director of the Department of Social Work Services of The Mount Sinai Hospital. He is also a recipient of the Ida M. Cannon Award of the Society of Social Work Directors of The American Hospital Association.

Opening Remarks

SIXTH DORIS SIEGEL MEMORIAL COLLOQUIUM
(APRIL 2, 1992)

On behalf of all the members of the Doris Siegel Memorial Fund Committee and the Colloquium Planning Committee, I am delighted to welcome you to the Sixth Doris Siegel Memorial Colloquium.

Doris was an inspirational leader who maintained a steadfast interest in delivering quality health care services, despite the ever present challenges of changing philosophies and demanding times. Today's program will describe the challenges before us as we confront the shift in health care services from a reliance on inpatient care to ambulatory care and its implications for health care providers and consumers.

Gary Rosenberg, PhD
Executive Secretary
The Doris Siegel Memorial Fund Committee

[Haworth co-indexing entry note]: "Opening Remarks." Rosenberg, Gary. Co-published simultaneously in *Social Work in Health Care* (The Haworth Press, Inc.) Vol. 20, No. 1, 1994, p. 1; and: *Social Work in Ambulatory Care: New Implications for Health and Social Services* (ed: Gary Rosenberg, and Andrew Weissman) The Haworth Press, Inc., 1994, p. 1. Multiple copies of this article/chapter may be purchased from The Haworth Document Delivery Center [1-800-3-HAWORTH; 9:00 a.m. - 5:00 p.m. (EST)].

Welcome

It is an honor for me to participate in this Sixth Doris Siegel Memorial Colloquium, my second.

The need for the kind of foresight, the vision that Doris Siegel had and still symbolizes is needed in times of change like we are now experiencing.

This colloquium addresses a timely topic–The Increasing Importance of Ambulatory Health Care Delivery Systems.

These changes are driven by major advances in medical care knowledge, technology, and skill and fueled by financial pressures from all governmental levels as well as private insurers.

What these changing patterns of health care delivery will mean for American health care policy, for patients and families, for all health care providers, and for our institutions of medical care, needs to be critically examined.

A Doris Siegel Colloquium seems like a good place to discuss these important ideas; the bringing together of various health care professionals to examine a critical issue is the hallmark of what Doris Siegel stood for–I wish you luck in your endeavors. Thank you.

John W. Rowe, MD
President
The Mount Sinai Medical Center

[Haworth co-indexing entry note]: "Welcome." Rowe, John W. Co-published simultaneously in *Social Work in Health Care* (The Haworth Press, Inc.) Vol. 20, No. 1, 1994, p. 3; and: *Social Work in Ambulatory Care: New Implications for Health and Social Services* (ed: Gary Rosenberg, and Andrew Weissman) The Haworth Press, Inc., 1994, p. 3. Multiple copies of this article/chapter may be purchased from The Haworth Document Delivery Center [1-800-3-HAWORTH; 9:00 a.m. - 5:00 p.m. (EST)].

The Sixth Doris Siegel Memorial Conference Tribute

Many of the people here today–to honor Doris Siegel–did not know her. Yet all of us who care about equality in care and professional standards are indebted to her.

It is over 20 years since Doris died. For some of us who worked with her, her presence is still fresh, and a couple of us talk to that presence from time to time. She combined drive, high standards, a hard work ethic, with an overall warmth and empathy. When she arrived at Mount Sinai in 1952, her directive was to professionalize the Department of Social Work Services. By 1966 the Department had academic standing in the new School of Medicine and in 1969, Doris occupied the first endowed Chair of Social Work in an American medical school. That is quite a track record.

Doris had opinions–which she firmly held–but she was also free and she "hung loose." If she brought a group together, a committee to plan, a staff to work with, she'd help them figure out their direction, firm it, and then would say "Go to it." Then it was yours, and she gave you the credit.

She was a lady with a mission. She drove herself to reach whatever goal she was supporting. During the period she worked here at Mount Sinai, it was up and down economically, yet even in the hard times she encouraged her staff to think program innovations and progress. She remained constant to her own ideals, which were to

---

[Haworth co-indexing entry note]: "The Sixth Doris Siegel Memorial Conference Tribute." Rehr, Helen. Co-published simultaneously in *Social Work in Health Care* (The Haworth Press, Inc.) Vol. 20, No. 1, 1994, pp. 5-6; and: *Social Work in Ambulatory Care: New Implications for Health and Social Services* (ed: Gary Rosenberg, and Andrew Weissman) The Haworth Press, Inc., 1994, pp. 5-6. Multiple copies of this article/chapter may be purchased from The Haworth Document Delivery Center [1-800-3-HAWORTH; 9:00 a.m. - 5:00 p.m. (EST)].

"reach out more aggressively not only to those we serve, but to those whom we should serve." She would have been very proud to be associated with Mount Sinai in the nineties–a decade in which Dr. John Rowe has committed Mount Sinai to its community–to "work closely with our neighbors to identify unmet health needs and respond with innovative programs."

Now, as then, change is not always welcomed by practitioners, administrators, even educators. Today we have various social and economic classes of care–separate care facilities are unequal–they foster racism and class differences, and one can assume that quality and services are different. A national health care program would at the least guarantee access to care for all. In Mount Sinai's proposed plan for reorganized ambulatory care, there would be one standard for all patients–irrespective of class, race or religion. Doris would be excited about these plans, which are not limited to clinic visits but include home care, long-term care and a guaranteed continuum of care. Primary, secondary and tertiary care would be available and merged across affiliated institutions and satellites. Our patients would be known to service centers in what Dr. Rowe has called a "translocation of service," into community care networks. This would meet Doris Siegel's dream for comprehensive continuity of care, reaching out into our many communities to find those in need and then integrating their care.

As constant as Doris was, she encouraged thinking and change. Her special gift was that she fostered trust in all those with whom she worked, and encouraged thinking about people and their needs.

I think today's panelists of the Sixth Doris Siegel Memorial Conference will demonstrate that even in these difficult times, innovative programs can be developed for today's and tomorrow's social-health needs.

These are Doris's ideals living on.

Helen Rehr, DSW Member
Doris Siegel Memorial Committee

PART 1:
INTRODUCTION

Social Work, the Family
and the Community

Gary Rosenberg, PhD

Mae West had been making silent films, using her body language to its best advantage. With the innovation of sound in film, she adapted her not-insignificant command of any setting and her flair for innuendo to her throaty voice, to her timing, and to her pointed delivery. In her first talking film, intent on watching a horse race at the track, she is beleaguered by a would-be gentleman suitor. "Ah, but for one touch of those delectable lips," he cries, "for just one kiss, I would give half my life." Unmoved by his supplications, Mae retorts in her inimitable drawl: "Why don't ya come up an' see me sometime. . . . I'll kiss ya ta-wice."

This story is something of a parable for social work in our current relationship with health care organizations. We have, in the years of

Gary Rosenberg is Executive Secretary for the Doris Siegel Memorial Fund Committee and Edith J. Baerwald Professor of Community Medicine (Social Work), Mount Sinai School of Medicine, City University of New York.

[Haworth co-indexing entry note]: "Social Work, the Family and the Community." Rosenberg, Gary. Co-published simultaneously in *Social Work in Health Care* (The Haworth Press, Inc.) Vol. 20, No. 1, 1994, pp. 7-20; and: *Social Work in Ambulatory Care: New Implications for Health and Social Services* (ed: Gary Rosenberg, and Andrew Weissman) The Haworth Press, Inc., 1994, pp. 7-20. Multiple copies of this article/chapter may be purchased from The Haworth Document Delivery Center [1-800-3-HAWORTH; 9:00 a.m. - 5:00 p.m. (EST)].

7

Reagan-Bush economics, become the supplicant suitor, whose value and resources for patient care have been kissed-off by the health care organization, as the survival needs of health care settings have been driven by DRGs, cost containment practices, and insurance reimbursement caps. Mae West's earthy wisdom holds another lesson for social work. She was able to transfer her dynamic body language to the dimension of sound in talking movies, in no way diminishing, but rather enhancing, the power and attraction of what she had to offer.

This brings us to the focus of this volume: the changing nature of health care in the next decade, with implications for social work with families. I want to address this issue: first, by talking about the changes in health care delivery; second, by reevaluating what we mean by "health"; and third, by describing the role of social work within health care institutions, within the community, and with families.

CHANGES IN HEALTH CARE DELIVERY

Cost containment, prospective payment procedures, DRGs and insurance reimbursement rates have impacted significantly on the nature of service delivery as well as on how long patients remain in an acute care facility. The U.S. has the lowest admission rates for acute care hospitals–U.S.-12.4%, Canada-13.3%, Germany-19.7%, coupled with the shortest length of stay of any major industrial country (Schwartz & Stanton, 1993). A number of services, formerly provided after admission, are now routinely provided on an out-patient, pre-admission basis. Physician group practices have capitalized on these services, often providing their own x-rays, lab work, ultrasound and scanning procedures (Burns, 1991). Freestanding ambulatory care facilities provide comparable diagnostic services. Technology has contributed to the de-institutionalizing of traditional hospital inpatient services. A large number of exploratory surgeries are now precluded by the use of magnetic resonance imaging. Further, consumer demand for accessible and affordable health care services has contributed to the growth in outpatient care.

Hospital-based ambulatory care facilities have increased revenue since 1985 by 123%, with the result that ambulatory care now accounts for nearly 25% of total patient revenue (Burns, 1991). These services include the operating room, radiology, laboratories, and physical therapy. Note that no mention is made of psychosocial support services in this area, despite the fact that such procedures, notably around diagnosis, can generate tremendous anxiety and depression in patients and families, contributing to illness and deterioration (Campbell, 1986). More about this later.

Despite this trend, since 1988, hospitals' share of outpatient revenue has declined nearly ten percent. Somebody else is appearing on the scene to provide these needed and wanted ambulatory services–physician group practices and free-standing diagnostic and laboratory facilities. Competition for service provision and the revenue that is generated comes also from the HMOs and managed care networks.

Between 1980 and 1989, hospital admissions plummeted from 36.1 million to 31.1 million, a decrease of 14%. If this current trend continues, and surely it will, projections suggest that there will be a 17% loss in inpatient admissions by the year 2000. More than half of dollars that employers spend on health care are now for outpatient services. The individual consumer, responsible for partial payment of his or her health care costs, is helped by this trend as well: charges for the same procedure can be up to 60% lower in an outpatient setting as compared with the cost of admission. Outpatient visits are up 40% in the last five years and are expected to increase another 106% by the year 2000. Ambulatory surgery now accounts for approximately 47% of all hospital surgeries. And finally, the average length of stay in 1989 was 5.51 days per admission. Driven by technological advances, government cost containment, insurance companies, and consumer demand, the essential acute care nature of traditional health care service delivery in hospital settings has changed.

The profits from outpatient services have been significant. Hospital administrators, seeking to downplay the inevitable shifts in health care from admissions to acute care facilities to ambulatory services, have tended to bury these significant profits in corporate overhead costs. In actuality, when fixed and overhead costs are properly allocated, a profit from between 15% and 20% can be anticipated from ambulatory care. Given these trends of the last 10 years, it is necessary to reevaluate the nature of ambulatory care services, their impact on the changed health care arena, and the evolving roles for the health care professions.

However, we must also consider the changing nature of the patients receiving health care. Physicians are no longer being looked to for what we called the cut, burn and poison approach to disease (surgery, radiation, and chemotherapy). People are looking for treatment and alleviation from pain, not necessarily to be cured; and they want to be involved in the course of their treatment. People are taking responsibility for their own health behavior. This phenomenon of personal accountability for individual health with an emphasis on prevention, not intervention has also spawned a concern for the community and the environment and its impact on health: a concern with smoking, nuclear power, lead poisoning, rodent control, asbestos, T.B., and immunizations and healthy eating habits. This surge within our culture toward individual involvement in one's own health care and community involvement in prevention is totally unlike our traditional emergency room, crisis-induced, physician-dependent perception of health care in which we grew up.

Further, there are more elderly in our population, and we are living longer. Statistically, the longer you live, the better your chances are for living even longer! In other words, if you are a female and live to be 60, you will probably live to be 86.5 years. If you live to be 80, you will probably live to be 91.3 years. And if you make it to 100, chances are you'll live to 103.6 (Society of Actuaries, 1983). The proportion of elderly in the general population is increasing; while with family size limitations, divorce rate, the impact of AIDS, and deferred parenthood, the proportion of youth is diminishing. Additionally, while comprising 12% of the American population, the elderly utilize the largest percentages of health care services: physician time, hospital admissions, medications sold. But this is the important fact here: their illnesses are less and less acute, and more and more chronic, extending over longer periods of their later years, and requiring a different nature of care than their parents before them who faced early, acute terminal illness and death. And people want to involve themselves in the course of their own treatment, at home, in the context of their families. Families are seen as the best "health insurance."

The shift in health care then, incurred by technological advances, by government cost regulation, by cultural changes in our perception of health, and by our own involvement in insuring health, is a paradigmatic one, from acute to chronic care. And the context of interventions, also incurred by government regulation, technological advances, and cultural demand, is from inpatient to ambulatory care. We are looking at a new and rapidly changing system of health care provision. And we are looking at health care and the meaning of health in our own lives from a totally different perspective than ever before.

If we think about the changes in health care in the next decade, we are looking at a predominance of ambulatory care services. We are also looking at an increasing population of chronic care patients: the elderly, persons with AIDS, and other patients with long-term illnesses that will, with advancing technology, be able to receive care in outpatient settings or in the home.

Secondly, we are on the threshold of a radically different approach to illness: one that integrates the biopsychosocial aspects of human life. The family systems social work practitioner is well trained and experienced in this process, and can lead the way in direct service, in facilitating practice-based research, in education, and in resource networking of community services. We can see the need for long-term biopsychosocial intervention with a large chronically ill patient population in non-traditional or home-based settings. Hospitals, as we have known them, will exist only for acute, episodic treatment of a critical nature.

Family care, both to enable caregiving to the identified patient and for contextual psychosocial intervention in the affective environment of the illness, can once again become a major domain of social work practice.

How will social work respond to the needs of families, to the health care institutions, and to the health needs of communities as we approach the twenty-first century? And how will we insure our own professional survival without incurring Mae West's kiss of death?

SOCIAL WORK IN THE YEAR 2000: THE FAMILY, THE INSTITUTION AND THE COMMUNITY

The Social Worker in the Family

Hans Falck (1988) suggests that the standards of practice and values inherent in our work are essentially social: i.e., the individual does not exist except in the context of his social environment. While this was the principle upon which the psychosocial approach to casework was established, it is not often reflected in the practice afforded in the health care setting. Yet, in practice, we tend to apply individualist strategies to our patients.

A study of data obtained from 350 social workers in 39 New England hospitals, found that workers perceived the primary problem affecting the patient's health in 27% of cases, to be the family. Yet the worker intervened in the family in only 7% of their caseloads. In the chronically ill elderly, a growing population of our concern, no intervention with family occurred in 52% of these cases (Carlton, Falck & Berkman, 1984). These figures are seriously disturbing. While we espouse a psychosocial approach to the treatment of patients, we practice a primarily illness-focused intervention, isolated and episodic in nature, and apparently without consequence to the integrated well-being of our patients.

What are some of the factors in understanding family reactions to chronic illness? We can enumerate a few: the family's stage of development in the life cycle; their sense of mastery and control over the illness; their previous experience with illness and the meaning attached to that history in their families of origin (Penn, 1983); the role of the illness in the function (or dysfunction) of the family (Schmidt, 1978; Caroff & Mailick, 1985); their cultural, ethnic, and religious beliefs and the impact of those beliefs on their understanding of the etiology of illness (Rolland, 1987). "Did God punish me with my child's cancer because of my infidelity?" Congruence among family members regarding the illness, its course, its treatment needs to be assessed (Weakland, 1977), as does triangulation or coalition-building which can militate against effective coping or interventions aimed at restructuring dysfunctional roles (Penn, 1983). Workers themselves can be unwittingly seduced into coalitions within the family as well (Leahey & Wright, 1985; Hoch & Hemmens, 1987).

If what the current literature identifies as psychosocial effects on physical illness are valid, then intervention in the family system must become a priority in the care of the chronically ill. The family should be recognized as the primary caregiving context of social work intervention.

As health care legislation will assuredly invoke family support systems to offset fiscal limitations, it will become increasingly essential to intervene directly within the family system itself, not only with the patient but within the caregiving context. When such caregiving or social support is unavailable, social work must also be equipped to intervene from within an institutional and community setting, integrating formal and informal systems of care.

Family Health Care and the Health Care Institution

As we expand our horizons to a biopsychosocial conceptualization, our services must mirror the redefinition of health and health care provision in the changing environment. An integrated approach to patient care will not only better address patient and family needs, but will greatly assist the health care organization in defining, developing, and sustaining its new role in the health care system of the next century.

The structural boundaries of the hospital should expand to an interactional linkage with other systems within the community. Social work administration can be the leader in delineating these inter-organizational linkages which will facilitate that integration. Such collaboration will result in a networking of services among various agencies in the community, with ongoing negotiation and integration of services among providers. As we view the casemix of the multi-faceted services provided in inpatient care, so we must begin to organize a "bundling" of services in outpatient chronic care: to include biomedical, legal, social, environmental and familial interventions from a variety of providers based in community practice.

The "bundling" or "packaging" of services can take a structured form, subsidized and organized by the hospital, viewed in this light as a center of community care. When the urban medical center commits to examining the possibilities of such partnerships with community agencies, it will often discover that it has already built a foundation of such relationships on which it can build new programs to meet the needs of the chronically ill.

Hospitals are changing and evolving community cooperative partnerships. Throughout the nation hospitals are trying to address the needs of specific community patient populations and their families. The Southeast Michigan AIDS Consortium reflects a collaboration of hospitals, home health providers, and insurance companies to develop methods of payment for uninsured patients with AIDS. A similar partnership in Pittsburgh established a maternal health program for substance abusing mothers and their children. A cooperative effort among Methodist Hospitals of Memphis and ten grammar schools has developed a nutrition education program and a children's cholesterol monitoring program (Davidson, 1992).

This kind of reconceptualization of our boundaries eliminates barriers to effective partnership, maximizes existing programs and creates opportunities for innovative approaches to the needs of families who cope with chronic illness. In doing this, we are essentially self-marketing: the community views us as the center of their health care and familial support needs (Rosenberg, Rehr & Blumenfield, 1993).

Family Health Care and the Community Agency

In order to address the needs of the community and patient, two major roles for social work may evolve: health promotion and wellness support in community service programs; and collaboration with families as partners in caregiving to the chronically ill.

This kind of support of the functional needs of our patients requires a significant shift in our approach to health care. If we are truly committed to the full spectrum of lifestyle intervention, then prevention and education are focal points for us to address. Empowering clients in their own health care is an essential component of this approach.

Community-based social work with families affords many advantages. We ease the burdens of care on family members; we empower them by enhancing choices in lifestyle activities and health care attention; we are in a position to intervene early in advance of acute distress, both with the patient and the family; we provide easier access to resources for the family; we reduce liability and risk for our own healthcare system; we address the fuller scope of health care which includes health as well as illness, integrating services from a wide spectrum of resources; and, simultaneously, and without too much effort, we market the viability of our services primarily by the effectiveness of what we offer.

Social Work and the Family Practice Team: Linking Formal Intervention with Informal Caregiving

In addition to hospital and community-based practice, services to families can be delivered by family medicine teams of physicians, nurse practitioners, and social workers. The social worker in this team setting is in a unique position to elaborate the notion of informal-formal partnerships between families and hospitals and between families and community agencies that have proven enormously helpful in easing the burden of caregivers to the chronically ill (Mayer, Kapust, Mulcahey, Helfand, Heinlein, Seltzer, Litchfield & Levin, 1990; Seltzer, Litchfield, Kapust & Mayer, 1992).

Education in the provision of case management tasks supplies the family caregiver with improved responses to her interactions with external resources, organizes and structures her own time, delimits the sense of helplessness by empowering her without pressuring her to relinquish control, provides her with resources according to her self-determined needs and wishes, and joins her in an egalitarian partnership with the caseworker, thereby supporting her and not intruding upon her own boundaries (Hoch & Hemmens, 1987; Lyman, 1989). Training the family member in case management, then, enables the caregiver to be more receptive to social work presence in the broader areas of psychosocial intervention (Seltzer, Ivry, & Lichtenfield, 1987).

Empowered in her own sphere of case management, the caregiver can afford to express her own dependency needs in the casework relationship. In this way, the social worker is also freed to alleviate the psychosocial components of illness in the overall family environment (Seltzer et al., 1992). Such collaboration between family and social worker does not exploit the family for its resources, but rather enhances them through education, appropriate service-provision, and essential psychosocial intervention (Brody, 1985).

When the caregiver is afforded sanction and approval for her efforts with her family member, she will probably have less need to aim for perfection in an overidealized quality of care. It's a paradoxical, but nonetheless authentic, intervention. More empowered, less alone, less guilty, and with the availability of a professional relationship where her own feelings can be explored, she can offer herself and her elderly parent a more authentic quality of loving care. When empathy is available for the resistance to "outside intervention," not only are the barriers lowered, but in doing so, the significant circumstances of isolation and guilt that contribute to family dysfunction are simultaneously alleviated (Montgomery & Borgatta, 1989).

Other members of the team can be supported in their functions by the presence of a social worker among them. The frequency and quality of exchanges between the physician and the patient can be enhanced; the services of the family practice can be more readily marketed through a social worker networking in the community; and she provides additional revenue-generating services to the practice (Greene, Kruse & Arthurs, 1985; Twersky & Cole, 1976).

Family Health Care and the Family Social Work Practitioner

The family social worker, increasingly perceived as a unique provider of essential services in the biopsychosocial treatment of chronic illness, can begin to market her services much as the private physician does his. As the physician is accountable to the health care system while functioning independently, so, too, the family practicing social worker must evolve toward a comparable role: independently self-directed, but accountable to the requirements and standards of care of the larger system.

Family service physicians are more keenly aware of the need for psychosocial intervention. But with ever-increasing caseloads, they too often resort to biophysical intervention with far less attention to the psychosocial aspects which they themselves espouse. Studies in Germany and the Netherlands evidence the willingness of family physicians to engage the private practice services of family social workers (Huygen & Smits, 1983). Note that I am not speaking about private psychotherapy practice. I am suggesting the viability of an innovative approach to family intervention practice by the individual practitioner, on a fee-for-service-basis.

Such a practitioner can intervene in families to which she is referred from a variety of sources: physicians; community agencies (including legal, political, educational, social, religious); and satisfied consumers. She can provide consultant and educational services regarding family dynamics in health care, as well as wellness and prevention services within the community. These services provide education in themselves while also serving to market her offerings. Provision of psychosocial family services in the primary care arena can serve as prevention for the evolution of more serious illness. When families are followed by the same worker over extended time, the dysfunctions so often erupting in tertiary care facilities for patient and for family can be arrested.

CONCLUSIONS

I hope my theme and that of the speakers at Sixth Doris Siegel Conference is clear: Social Work needs to reclaim its early focus on community health and continue to develop its expertise in the provision of clinical services for individuals and families facing the complex decisions about values and lifestyles necessitated by advances in health related technology and information.

REFERENCES

Albert, S.M., Litvin, S.J., Kleban, M.H., & Brody, E.M. (1991). Caregiving daughters' perceptions of their own and their mothers' personalities. *The Gerontologist*, 31(4), 476-482.

Anderson, R.E. & Carter, I. (1978). *Human behavior in the social environment: A social systems approach* (2nd edition). New York: Aldine Publishing.

Bowen, M. (1960). A family concept of schizophrenia. In D. Jackson (Ed.). *The etiology of schizophrenia* (pp. 346-372). New York: Basic Books.

Brody, E. (1985). Parent care as a normative family stress. *The Gerontologist*, 25 (1), 19-29.

Burns, L.A. (1991). Financial issues in ambulatory care. *Top Health Care Finance*, 17(3), 53-65.

Calabrese, J.R., Kling, M.S., & Gold, P.W. (1987). Alterations in immunocompetence during stress, bereavement, and depression: Focus on neuroendocrine regulation. *American Journal of Psychiatry,* 144(9), 1123-1134.

Campbell, T. (1986). Family's impact on health: A critical review. *Family Systems Medicine,* 4(2&3), 135-200.

Carlton, T.O., Falck, H.S., & Berkman, B. (1984). The use of theoretical constructs and research data to establish a base for clinical social work in health settings. *Social Work in Health Care,* 10(2), 27-40.

Caroff, P. & Mailick, M.D. (1985). The patient has a family: Reaffirming social work's domain. *Social Work in Health Care,* 10(4), 17-34.

Cassileth, B.R., Lusk, E.J., Miller, D.S., Brown, L.L., & Miller, C. (1985). Psychosocial correlates of survival in advanced malignant disease? *New England Journal of Medicine,* 312(24), 1551-1555.

Davidson, D. (1992, January 20). A decade of competition ends–a new era of cooperation begins. *Hospitals,* pp. 44-50.

Estes, C.L. & Binney, E.A. (1989). The biomedicalization of aging: Dangers and dilemmas. *The Gerontologist,* 29(5), 587-596.

Falck, H.S. (1988). *Social work: The membership perspective.* New York: Springer Publishing Co.

Gallagher, D., Rose, J., Rivera, P., Lovett, S., & Thompson, L.W. (1989). Prevalence of depression in family caregivers. *The Gerontologist,* 29(4), 449-456.

Gambe, R. & Getzel, G.S. (1989). Group work with gay men with AIDS. *Social Casework,* 70, 172-179.

Gonzalez, S., Steinglass, P., & Reiss, D. (1989). Putting the illness in its place: Discussion groups for families with chronic medical illnesses. *Family Process,* 11, 457-486.

Greene, G., Kruse, K.A., & Arthurs, R.J. (1985). Family practice social work: A new area of specialization. *Social Work in Health Care,* 10(3), 53-73.

Grolnick, L. (1972). A family perspective of psychosomatic factors in illness: A review of the literature. *Family Process,* 11, 457-486.

Hoch, C., & Hemmens, G.C. (1987). Linking informal and formal help: Conflict along the continuum of care. *Social Service Review,* 61, 432-446.

Huygen, F.J.A. & Smits, A.J.A. (1983). Family therapy, family somatics, and family medicine. *Family Systems Medicine,* 1(1), 23-32.

Irwin, M., Daniels, M., Bloom, E.T., Smith, T.L., & Weiner, H. (1987). Life events, depressive symptoms, and immune function. *American Journal of Psychiatry,* 144(4), 437-442.

Jarrett, W.H. (1985). Caregiving within kinship systems: Is affection really necessary? *The Gerontologist,* 25(1), 5-10.

Johnson, H.C. (1991). Theories of Kernberg and Kohut: Issues of scientific validation. *Social Service Review,* 65(3), 403-433.

Johnston, M., Martin, M., & Gumaer, J. (1992). Long-term parental illness and children: Perils and promises. *School Counselor,* 39(3), 225-231.

Leahey, M. & Wright, L.M. (1985). Intervening with families with chronic illness. *Family Systems Medicine,* 3(1), 60-69.

Littlefield, C.H. & Rushton, J.W. (1986). When a child dies: The sociology of bereavement. *Journal of Personality and Social Psychology*, 51(4), 797-802.

Lyman, K.A. (1989). Bringing the social back in: A critique of the biomedicalization of dementia. *The Gerontologist*, 29(5), 597-605.

Manne, S.L. & Zautra, A.J. (1989). Spouse criticism and support: Their association with coping and psychological adjustment among women with rheumatoid arthritis. *Journal of Personality and Social Psychology*, 56(4), 608-617.

Mayer, J.B., Kapust, L.R., Mulcahey, A.L., Helfand, L., Seltzer, M.M., Litchfield, L.C., & Levin, R.J. (1990). Empowering families of the chronically ill: A partnership in a hospital setting. *Social Work in Health Care*, 14(4), 73-90.

Meissner, W.W. (1966). Family dynamics and psychosomatic processes. *Family Process*, 5, 142-161.

Minuchin, S., Rosman, B.L., & Baker, L. (1978). *Psychosomatic Families*. Cambridge, MA: Harvard University.

Montgomery, R.J.V. & Borgatta, E.F. (1989). The effects of alternative support strategies on family caregiving. *The Gerontologist*, 29(4), 457-464.

Paterson, G.W. (1987). Managing grief and bereavement. *Primary Care*, 14(2), 403-415.

Peck, B.B. (1975). Physical medicine and family dynamics: The dialectics of rehabilitation. *Family Process*, 13(4), 469-480.

Penn, P. (1983). Coalitions and binding interactions in families with chronic illness. *Family Systems Medicine*, 1(2), 16-25.

Richardson, H.B. (1945). *Patients have families*. New York: Commonwealth Fund.

Rolland, J.S. (1987). Family illness paradigms: Evolution and significance. *Family Systems Medicine*, 5(4), 482-503.

Rose-Itkoff, C. (1987). Lupus: An interactional approach. *Family Systems Medicine*, 5(3), 313-321.

Rosenberg, G., Rehr, H., & Blumenfield, S. (1992). Community partnerships in the 1990's. *Mt. Sinai Hospital Journal of Medicine*, 59(6), 479-486.

Sacks, O. (1993). Narrative and medicine. *Mt. Sinai Hospital Journal of Medicine*, 60(2), 127-131.

Schmidt, D.D. (1978). The family as the unit of medical care. *Journal of Family Practice*, 7(2), 303-313.

Schmidt, D.D. (1983). Family determinants of disease: Depressed lymphocyte function following the loss of a spouse. *Family Systems Medicine*, 1(1), 33-39.

Schwartz, L.L. & Stanton, M.W. (1993). We'll need those excess hospital beds [letter to the editor]. *The New York Times*, p. A16.

Seltzer, M.M., Ivry, J., & Lichtenfield, L.C. (1987). Family members as case managers: Partnership between the formal and informal support networks. *The Gerontologist*, 27(6), 722-728.

Seltzer, M.M., Litchfield, L.C., Kapust, L.R., & Mayer, J.B. (1992). Professional and family collaboration in case management: A hospital-based replication of a community-based study. *Social Work in Health Care*, 17(1), 1-22.

Smith, G.C., Smith, M.F., & Toseland, R.W. (1991). Problems identified by family caregivers in counseling. *The Gerontologist*, 31(1), 15-22.

Society of Actuaries (1993). *Group annuity mortality table.*

Stuifbergen, A.K. (1987). The impact of chronic illness on families. *Family and Community Health*, 9(4), 43-51.

Subramanian, K. & Rose, S.D. (1988). Social work and the treatment of chronic pain. *Health and Social Work*, 13(1), 49-60.

Sullivan, D.H., Gramm, T., & Hetzer, P. (1990). Ambulatory care for patients with acute leukemia: An alternative to frequent hospitalization. *Journal of Professional Nursing*, 6(5), 300-309.

Toseland, R.W., Rossiter, C.M., & Labrecque, M.S. (1989). Group interventions to support family caregivers: A review and analysis. *The Gerontologist*, 29(4), 438-448.

Twersky, R.K. & Cole, W.M. (1976). Social work fees in medical care: A review of the literature and report of a survey. *Social Work in Health Care*, 2(1), 77-84.

Weakland, J.H. (1977). "Family somatics"–a neglected edge. *Family Process*, 16, 263-272.

Zarit, S.H. & Toseland, R.W. (1989). Current and future direction in family caregiving research. *The Gerontologist*, 29(4), 481-483.

Zisook, S., DeVaul, R.A., & Click, M.A. (1982). Measuring symptoms of grief and bereavement. *American Journal of Psychiatry*, 139(12), 1590-1593.

Zola, I.K. (1972). Medicine as an institution of social control. *Sociological Review*, 20, 487-504.

PART 2:
PRESENTATIONS

The New York City Health System: A Paradigm Under Siege

Ronda Kotelchuck, MRP

INTRODUCTION

Thank you for inviting me to be here today. First, let me preface the comments I will make this afternoon.

I was asked to discuss the implications of the shift to ambulatory care from the perspective of the consumer. I am going to do that particularly from the perspective of the low income consumer–the consumer with the fewest choices and the most limited access. I am going to do this for two reasons: first, because it is the group that the Health & Hospitals Corporation primarily serves, and the group that I know the most about, and second, because the experience of low income consumers highlights and presents an intensified version of the problems of the system that are faced to varying degrees by all.

Ronda Kotelchuck is Executive Director of the Primary Care Development Corporation, New York, NY 10007.

[Haworth co-indexing entry note]: "The New York City Health System: A Paradigm Under Siege." Kotelchuck, Ronda. Co-published simultaneously in *Social Work in Health Care* (The Haworth Press, Inc.) Vol. 20, No. 1, 1994, pp. 21-33; and: *Social Work in Ambulatory Care: New Implications for Health and Social Services* (ed: Gary Rosenberg, and Andrew Weissman) The Haworth Press, Inc., 1994, pp. 21-33. Multiple copies of this article/chapter may be purchased from The Haworth Document Delivery Center [1-800-3-HAWORTH; 9:00 a.m. - 5:00 p.m. (EST)].

21

Second, I am really going to focus on the shift between models of care–inpatient, tertiary care on the one hand and primary and preventive care on the other. Whether acute, tertiary care is given in the hospital or out is not the critical or interesting issue in my mind. The critical and interesting issue is the kind of care that is given, its content and approach, the model or paradigm that it represents.

Finally, I am going to make several arguments this afternoon. First, I am going to argue that health services, like health itself, exist on a spectrum and that to be efficient and effective, this spectrum must be balanced and its services coordinated. I will argue that services in New York City's health system are neither balanced nor coordinated; that instead, they are dominated by an acute, tertiary, inpatient model of care; and that much as we would like to think otherwise, they have not shifted toward non-acute models of care over the last two decades. Rather, the opposite has occurred. And the result, particularly for the low income consumer, has been disastrous. The result is that services are unavailable, utterly inappropriate to need and exorbitantly expensive. Finally, I will argue that, for the first time, there are signs that a change may be in the offing.

THE SPECTRUM OF HEALTH SERVICES

Just like health status, health care services exist on a spectrum. That spectrum begins with public health and preventive care–measures that are not even necessarily framed as health services nor oriented to individuals. Yet over the past they have proven to be the single most effective means of improving the health of the public.

The spectrum continues with primary care, where the first encounter and the vast majority of all interactions between the patient and the medical system take place. Here the objective is health maintenance, early detection and intervention before the disease process has progressed and while illness is easy and inexpensive to treat.

The spectrum then progresses to include acute inpatient care–care that is appropriate when the patient is intensely ill and needs intensive intervention. Acute care is institutionally-based and expensive. It is a model that is increasingly high technology, highly-specialized and academic in its orientation.

The spectrum continues, for those who are not acutely ill but who cannot be self-sufficient, with long-term care–both institutionally-based nursing home care and community-based home health care and supportive services. These services may be short term and recuperative or long-term and custodial in nature.

To operate efficiently and effectively, both in terms of meeting human need and optimal resource use, all of these services must be balanced and coordinated and the patient must be able to move quickly to the level that is most appropriate to his or her need.

A SPECTRUM OUT OF BALANCE

First, I would like to argue that the New York City health system is not a balanced one. It is a system dominated by a single model of care–acute, tertiary care medicine, and that both ends of the spectrum–primary and preventive care and aftercare care–are woefully underdeveloped. The results are services that are inappropriate to need–particularly the burgeoning health care needs of low income consumers;–services that are utilized inappropriately; and services that are extraordinarily costly. Why is the acute, tertiary care model of medicine so dominant in New York City?

Academic Medicine. One possible answer lies in the fact that New York is the world capital of academic medicine, and academic medicine has focused on highly specialized, tertiary services to the neglect of other models of care. New York City and its environs are the home of seven medical schools. Graduate medical education is an export industry. With barely three percent of the nation's population, New York City trains over 15 percent of the nation's doctors. Three-quarters of its 75 hospitals are teaching hospitals and teaching intensity–measured by the ratio of residents to workload–is 40 percent higher in New York City than the average in the nation's other large urban areas.

Very few of the young doctors that New York trains, however, are headed for careers in primary care. Fully 70 percent go into subspecialties; only 30 percent go into primary care specialties–general internal medicine, pediatrics, obstetrics or family practice. This distribution is precisely the opposite of what is considered an optimal balance. In Canada 50 percent of physicians practice primary care; in the United Kingdom 70 percent do. New York's record in family practice is even more dismal. Only five percent of medical graduates go into family practice in New York City, compared to a national average of 15 percent.

In spite of the need, a growing recognition of the importance of primary care, and a growing rhetoric, the shift among young doctors entering the profession appears to be away from primary care. A recent *New England Journal of Medicine* article found that between 1986 and 1991 the number of medical school graduates selecting careers in primary care fell by 19 percent.[1]

The Payment System. The second and more fundamental explanation of the shape of New York's health system lies in its payment system. I firmly believe that we get what we pay for, and we are paying for a very strong acute, tertiary care system. Conversely, we do not pay for the alternatives, and thus they cannot grow or develop.

Health care finance and coverage are built on an insurance model, originally developed by Blue Cross and commercial carriers and later adopted by Medicare and Medicaid. The insurance model deals well with risk–the risk of unlikely but expensive, catastrophic events. It was never meant to deal with certainty. Thus, if you rely on traditional health insurance, chances are that you have excellent inpatient, acute care coverage. In fact, 71 percent of premium costs in New York go to cover inpatient expenses. Chances are that your greatest out-of-pocket cost occurs when you want to visit your doctor. And to be paid for a physical exam, a well child visit or a screening mammogram, you must feign illness. The use of expensive inpatient and acute services is a risk. The need for prevention, health maintenance and primary care is a certainty. The need for maternity care among young women is a certainty. Dependency and chronic illness among the elderly is a certainty. And these services are covered poorly, if at all, by the insurance system.

If you are a low income consumer and you rely on Medicaid, which was patterned after the insurance system, ironically the payment bias toward acute, inpatient care and against primary care is even stronger. Only four percent of all Medicaid dollars are spent on primary care, compared to 33 percent on inpatient acute care and 40 percent on long-term care. Although inpatient rates have been highly controlled, until very recently Medicaid paid hospitals at cost, and those costs have been increased each year to account for inflation and a variety of other factors. Consider how rates for primary care and outpatient care have been treated by comparison:

Medicaid fees for private physicians have been frozen virtually since its inception in the mid-1960s. Today Medicaid pays a private physician an average of $11 a visit. Have any of you tried offering your physician $11 recently? If so, you learned what Medicaid patients know instinctively. Physicians, even those wanting to serve Medicaid clients, cannot possibly make a living, except by running a "mill," and by now the rates have fallen so low that most Medicaid mills are now an endangered species.

New York's low income patients have been forced to rely instead on far more expensive outpatient departments and emergency rooms for their routine care. In contrast to private physicians, Medicaid paid at cost for outpatient department and emergency room care until 1981 when, in an effort to control costs, it froze these rates at $60 per visit. Medicaid now pays $65 plus the cost of capital for an outpatient visit, while the actual cost in hospitals across the City has risen to an average of twice that amount. Outpatient clinics have now become the single largest source of financial loss to New York City's hospitals, and many hospitals are moving to reduce outpatient services and the financial liability that results.

What about other primary care alternatives? Ten community health centers serve New Yorkers, down from 15 during the 1960s and 1970s, and provide an important source of community-based primary care. While paid equitably by Medicaid, they are heavily reliant on federal Section 330 for funds to cover the uninsured and the National Health Service Corps for physicians. Section 330 monies have been seriously cut back and diverted to non-urban areas while funding of the National Health Service Corps virtually dried up during the 1980s.

At the far end of the spectrum is public health and preventive health services, such as lead poisoning, rodent control, immunization, school health, the screening and control of TB and sexually transmitted diseases. These are entirely omitted from the insurance/third party coverage rubric, and are dependent instead on categorical, public funding. The 1980s saw radical cutbacks in funding of such programs at the federal level, with responsibility devolving largely to states and localities. Now, faced with a major fiscal crisis at these levels, the City has been largely forced to abandon its commitment to public and preventive health as well.

Finally, at the opposite end of the spectrum, long-term care has also traditionally been omitted from the insurance rubric. Because Medicaid pays for long-term care, it has become the insurer by default, not just for poor but for middle income patients who either transfer their assets to become eligible or quickly impoverish themselves enough to qualify. Fully half of all Medicaid dollars in New York State go for the provision of long-term care.

Medicaid has paid largely at cost for long-term care. In order to control the program, however, the State froze the building of new nursing home capacity for nearly 20 years. In the mid-1980s, the State finally lifted the freeze, but replaced it instead with limits on reimbursable construction costs that were so stringent as to make building in New York City unfeasible.

THE CONSEQUENCES OF AN UNBALANCED SYSTEM

What are the consequences of the system we have paid for, particularly for the low income consumer? The consequences are (1) the absence of services appropriate to meet the bulk of health care needs; (2) the forced over-reliance of the poor on needlessly expensive and inappropriate acute and tertiary care oriented services, to the point that these are overutilized and their access is in jeopardy; (3) the inability to address growing health care needs with severe compromises in health and human life; and (4) a cost escalation which cannot be contained because it is integral to and generated by the very model of care offered.

The Absence of Appropriate and Needed Services. Because of low Medicaid fees, private physicians have virtually abandoned low income communities over the last 20 years. Today, poor people simply do not have the option of seeing a private physician in the community.

To document this abandonment, in 1989 the Community Service Society surveyed physicians practicing in nine low income communities in New York City which are home to 1.7 million New Yorkers.[2] The survey initially identified 702 physicians practicing in these communities. To identify physicians practicing genuine primary care and who were truly available to the community, they factored out physicians who did not have admitting privileges, who did not treat Medicaid patients, who were over the age of 65, who did not practice more than 20 hours a week and who did not offer 24-hour telephone access. When they did this, they discovered that *only 28 physicians were available to serve the primary care needs of 1.7 million low income New Yorkers.*

Over-Reliance on Inappropriate and Expensive Services. Patients have instead been forced to turn to far more expensive, institutionally-based outpatient and emergency room services. Outpatient services are largely organized to reflect the needs of teaching residents, the majority of whom are seeking careers in subspecialty medicine. Thus, outpatient clinics function effectively to produce patients with a particular malady in one place at one time, often in a single block instead of by individual appointment. For the patient, care is anything but efficient and effective. OPDs are large, fragmented, chaotic, and specialty-oriented. Care entails hours of waiting and there is no semblance of a physician-patient relationship or continuity of care or frequently the presence of medical records.

Emergency rooms are organized to provide intensive, life-saving emergency intervention. Yet because by law they must treat patients and they are available 24-hours-a-day, ERs have increasingly become the only access to care available. The Health & Hospitals Corporation estimates that half of all emergency room visits are for conditions that could and should be treated in primary care settings. A recent study of non-emergency use of the City's Emergency Medical System by New York University's Wagner School found lack of primary care at fault. "Forty five percent of the callers said they would not have called EMS if they could have talked to a physician at the time of the problem. Forty seven percent had no regular source of primary health care."[3]

Without an infrastructure available to prevent illness or to identify and intervene in its early stages, patients' first encounter with the health system is often the emergency room when they are in the advanced and life-threatening stages of illness. At this point there is no choice. Massive, intense and expensive intervention is required and given. Known as the practice of "resurrection medicine," health care needs are neglected until patients are at death's doorstep and then the medical system rushes in, sparing nothing, to bring them back to life and then return them to the circumstances that produced the illness.

Lack of appropriate services forces a similar overuse of inpatient care. A growing body of work documenting unnecessary use of inpatient services has been authored by John Billings.[4] He identified a set of "ambulatory care sensitive" (ACS) conditions such as diabetes, hypertension, asthma, respiratory infections and otitis media which, if properly managed on an ambulatory care basis, should rarely require hospitalization. He found admissions for these conditions to be "exponentially related to income." Admission rates for ACS conditions were three times higher among Medicaid patients (35.2 admissions/1000 population) than among non-Medicaid populations (9.6 admissions). And while ACS admission rates were stable for non-Medicaid populations, they are growing significantly for Medicaid patients.

While the work on ACS conditions adds to our understanding of the inappropriateness of health services as they are currently configured, it is a new rendition of an old phenomena of perfectly preventable conditions that end up exacting an enormous and needless toll in terms of human suffering as well as resources. These include low birth weight and premature infants whose condition can be prevented by education, nutrition and prenatal care; measles which has reached epidemic proportions despite a vaccine that can prevent it entirely and a host of other conditions.

The Inability to Address Growing Health Care Needs. The inappropriateness of services has never been more clear than over the last four years during which the health status of New Yorkers has seriously deteriorated. Called by some a "health quake," a set of major epidemics has besieged New York City's poor communities in particular, aided and abetted, if not directly caused by dramatic growth in poverty, homelessness and medical indigency. And New York's health system, without an infrastructure of public, preventive and primary care services, has been helpless to intervene.

1. New York City is the epicenter of AIDS and HIV illness in the nation. Fully one-quarter of the nation's AIDS patients reside in New York. Since the epidemic began 37,000 New Yorkers have

been diagnosed with AIDS and 24,000 have died. Increasingly those cases are located among the City's poor and minority populations. Never has early detection and intervention been more important than in a person whose immune system is compromised and for whom every infection is a life threatening one.

2. Drug abuse has become the second major epidemic, fueled by the use of the cheap, widely available and highly addictive cocaine derivative, crack. There are an estimated 200,000 narcotics users (mostly heroin) and 400,000 non-narcotics (cocaine and crack) users in New York City. Despite the soaring toll on foster care, welfare, shelter, health care, police and the courts, the City offers only 40,000 drug treatment slots to stem this epidemic.

The health effects of growing drug use, aside from the spread of AIDS, are many in number, devastating in nature and overwhelming to New York City's health system. Births to drug abusing women increased 437 percent between 1981 and 1988, and drug use has contributed singularly to growing neonatal illness. A newborn exposed to drugs is 4.4 times more likely to be low birthweight, 4.0 times more likely to be admitted to a neonatal ICU and 1.6 times more likely to die in the first year. Drug use has brought a variety of other health consequences. The number of psychiatric inpatients using drugs rose 70.3 percent from 1985 to 1989, while among medical, obstetrical and pediatric patients, those using drugs rose 67 percent.

3. Tuberculosis is the most recent and perhaps most alarming epidemic, because it is increasingly drug-resistant and everyone is at risk. After decades of decline, TB rates rose steadily during the 1980s, doubling between 1980 to 1989. In the following year, however, it soared by 38 percent.

4. At epidemic levels are a variety of other illnesses as well—sexually transmitted diseases, other infectious and respiratory diseases, mental illness, violence and trauma. However, no measure captures overall health status better than excess mortality—deaths which would not have occurred if the New York City experience paralleled the rest of the nation. Excess deaths rose 522 percent, from 890 deaths in 1985 to 5,805 in 1988. In 1985 excess deaths comprised one percent of total deaths; by 1988 they had risen to over eight percent. Nor have rising death rates visited the City's

population equally. Hardest hit are young adults, age 25 to 44, normally the healthiest group in the prime of their productive and child-bearing years. Similarly, the plague is highly localized among low income and minority New Yorkers. Well-known is the study by McCord and Freeman that found the rate of male survival over the age of 40 to be higher in Bangladesh than it is in Harlem today.

Without a well-developed infrastructure providing public, primary and preventive health services, New York's health system has been helpless to stem these epidemics. Instead, these patients have appeared, desperately ill, in New York's emergency rooms and required intensive, inpatient acute care. The result, particularly during 1989 and 1990, has been overcrowding of New York's inpatient services, compounded by the consequences of an underdeveloped aftercare system. With nursing homes running at 99 percent occupancy many hospital patients, no longer needing acute care but unable to be self-sufficient, cannot be discharged. So ironically, patients inappropriately occupy badly needed acute care beds, where they cannot receive the therapeutic and recuperative services they need, making those beds unavailable in turn to dozens of patients who wait for hours and sometimes for days in emergency rooms for admission.

The result, particularly from 1988 through 1990, has been the health system equivalent of gridlock, where traffic cannot be diverted before reaching the intersection nor can it be speeded through the intersection, so it stalls, paralyzing the least appropriate and most expensive service on the spectrum.

HOPEFUL SIGNS?

The acute, tertiary care paradigm is breaking down. For advocates of primary care, there are hopeful signs of growing support for another.

At the federal level, Medicare has just moved to a new fee schedule that rewards primary care specialties at the expense of surgical and subspecialty physicians. The importance and effectiveness of community health centers in meeting the needs of low income communities are beginning to be recognized. Appropriations for Section 330, which supports community health centers, are increasing for the first time in nearly a decade and the feds have created a new category of federally-qualified health centers where Medicaid will pay for services at full cost. Similarly, after being virtually defunded, monies are once more being pumped into the National Health Service Corps, which places physicians and other health professionals in underserved communities.

At the State level there are similar signs. In the first breakthrough since the late 1970s, the Medicaid program has begun to enhance fees for private physicians serving children, provided they meet primary care criteria. Similarly, Medicaid over the last three years has structured incentives for primary care management into reimbursement of prenatal services through the PCAP program and AIDS care through the five-tier rate system. The State has also created a state-subsidized primary care insurance program for children. And recently, the State decided to weight Medicaid reimbursement of hospital medical education costs to significantly favor primary care residencies.

Medicaid Managed Care. But the most potentially significant development has been enactment of the Medicaid Managed Care Program. Last Spring the Legislature passed a bill requiring that within five years half of all Medicaid recipients be enrolled in managed care. Instead of paying fee-for-service whenever the patient utilizes a service, under managed care Medicaid will pay a flat sum to an HMO or managed care plan to provide a comprehensive set of Medicaid inpatient and outpatient services. The HMO or plan keeps the surplus if it can reduce the cost of services needed to less than the premium it receives. Similarly, it is at financial risk if the patient requires services costing more than the premium.

Medicaid managed care is a major change in payment policy with major potential for moving the system toward primary care.

- Effectively, through managed care, Medicaid has decided to purchase a new and different product for its clients. Instead of passively paying for fragmented services, Medicaid has decided that it will purchase a package of coordinated, comprehensive services for each client. Instead of purchasing these from providers, Medicaid will make one party–the HMO or plan–responsible.

- Primary care providers should take front and center stage under managed care, since they play a key role in maintaining and preserving the patient's health and serving as gatekeeper to the more expensive services. New York State's program requires that participating primary care providers meet a set of baseline standards. They must be licensed and Board certified or eligible, assure continuity of care, have inpatient admitting privileges, offer 24-hour telephone coverage, and provide a minimum of five sessions per week.
- Managed care shifts the heart of the system, not to mention the flow of funds, from providers, most notably acute care institutions, to HMOs or plans. Acting as insurers and new third party payors, these parties will presumably seek the balance of services needed for the best price available.
- Finally and most importantly, managed care at last makes possible a viable funding stream for primary care physicians. The HMO or plan generally contracts for primary, specialty and acute care services and is free to allocate funds among these providers in any manner it sees fit, thus removing for the first time the iron curtain that traditionally separates inpatient, acute care funding from ambulatory care.

But in tandem with its progressive potential, managed care also poses potential danger to Medicaid clients, depending on how the program is implemented.

Managed care is built on a financial incentive to limit services. Expensive services can be reduced through the provision of good primary and preventive care and good medical management, or they can simply be denied through an elaborate system of required authorizations and reviews. The threat looms all the more real, since under a soon-to-be mandatory system, the Medicaid clients will no longer be able to vote their choice with their feet.

Whether Medicaid managed care, like the nascent changes in primary care payment policy at the State and federal level, can be orchestrated into a genuine shift away from the acute care paradigm rests in our hands, among others.

The 1990s will be a time of crucial opportunity for those of us dedicated to building a health system that reflects and responds to the entire range of health needs experienced by all New Yorkers and indeed all Americans. The rising costs and the growing threat of medical indigency are now feeding a movement for national health reform. We must assure that the debate is not limited to different methods of finance but goes to the heart of the model of care delivered. Unless it accomplishes this, national health reform will be utterly incapable of addressing the attendant issues of cost and access.

Thank you.

REFERENCES

1. Jack M. Colwill, M.D., "Where Have All the Primary Care Applicants Gone?" *New England Journal of Medicine*, Vol. 326, No. 6, Feb. 6, 1992, pp. 387-393.

2. Christel Brellochs, Angjean Carter, Barbara Caress and Amy Goldman, *Building Primary Health Care Services in New York City's Low-Income Communities*, Community Service Society of New York, NY, NY, 1990.

3. James R. Knickman, "Improving Ambulance Service in New York City," *Early Findings*, Robert F. Wagner Graduate School of Public Service Health Research Program, NY, NY. March 1992.

4. John Billings, cited in *One Policy, Fifty-Eight Results: An Update on Variation in Hospitalization Rates of Medicaid Clients in New York State*, NYS Association of Counties, State Communities Aid Association, January 2, 1992.

Community Based Care: The New Health Social Work Paradigm

June Simmons, MSW

INTRODUCTION

The American health care system is undergoing a profound transformation caused in part by changes in health care needs and new technology. As more people are kept alive with chronic medical conditions, health care is shifting from an acute care and episodic focus to an extended care, continuity-based focus as eighty percent of morbidity and ninety percent of mortality are now due to chronic conditions.[1] While health care was previously centered in the physician's office and the acute care hospital, it has expanded to involve a complex array of community-based care providers. Thus, a significant emerging concern is the coordination of health care services provided to individuals through a multitude of health care providers and settings. This is an important emerging area of social work program development.

This article explores the shift of health care to primary and community care settings and the implications for the delivery of health social work.

June Simmons is Executive Vice President of the Visiting Nurse Association of Los Angeles, 520 South Lafayette Park Place, Suite 500, Los Angeles, CA 90057.

[Haworth co-indexing entry note]: "Community Based Care: The New Health Social Work Paradigm." Simmons, June. Co-published simultaneously in *Social Work in Health Care* (The Haworth Press, Inc.) Vol. 20, No. 1, 1994, pp. 35-46; and: *Social Work in Ambulatory Care: New Implications for Health and Social Services* (ed: Gary Rosenberg, and Andrew Weissman) The Haworth Press, Inc., 1994, pp. 35-46. Multiple copies of this article/chapter may be purchased from The Haworth Document Delivery Center [1-800-3-HAWORTH; 9:00 a.m. - 5:00 p.m. (EST)].

THE SHIFTING LOCUS OF HEALTH CARE

During much of this century, the hospital has been the site of the largest health care expenditures and the user of the major proportion of health care resources. Over the last two decades, several factors have forced hospitals to change their focus from inpatient services to the broader continuum of health care services. These changes began with the appreciable rise of medical technology, the dissatisfaction with the medical profession's explanation of the occurrences of various treatments for similar conditions, and with the varying lengths of stay of patients in the hospital with similar conditions around the country. The introduction of the prospective payment system (DRGs) for Medicare patients intensified the pressures on the hospitals to change.

Secondly, there has been an increasing utilization of outpatient and community-based services–outpatient care, ambulatory surgery, emergency services, home health care, nursing homes and specialty rehabilitation centers. Thirdly, patients within the acute care hospital setting are increasingly very ill, with complex and highly technical needs. Inpatient hospital beds are increasingly being used for intensive care. Fourthly, since the early 1980s, hospital admissions have declined despite a growing number of elderly people who were traditionally high users of inpatient acute-care resources. Finally, the length of time a patient spends in the hospital continues to decrease dramatically. This trend has been supported by the growing availability and increasing use of sophisticated technology, which has made it possible for major diagnosis and treatment activities to move to the physician's office and other community care settings.[2]

THE LOCUS OF SOCIAL WORK SERVICES

For most of its history, health care social work has been primarily based in the inpatient hospital setting. The location, nature and funding for these services have been directly tied to the design and financing arrangements of the health care system. And although the hospital will remain a significant force, pivotal social work services, as has happened in medical services, will move out of the inpatient setting and into outpatient departments, physicians offices, community and in-home settings.

With a smaller proportion of patients being cared for in the hospital setting and with patients having increasingly brief stays during which they are extremely sick, the primary locus of health care social work must change. The inpatient hospital will not continue to be the primary funding base for the provision of health related social work services.

Funding strategies to shift support for social work to ambulatory care practice settings become crucial as these settings emerge as a dominant site for provision of care. Outpatient and community-based care costs now account for more than fifty percent of dollars employers spend on health care. Outpatient services have almost tripled over the last half of the 1980s; ambulatory surgery now accounts for fifty percent of all hospital-based surgery.[3]

People with chronic health conditions need care and support over longer periods of time. In the new world of health care they will be receiving that care in a variety of places. Coordinating mechanisms should be developed to assure continuity and appropriate provision of these health care services. Social work leadership in the design and delivery of health care coordination services is crucial to the future role of social work in health care.

As we move from specific diagnosis-focused interventions to broader systems of care that emphasize continuing support over the life of the patients' health conditions, additional social work program development roles emerge. These include health promotion, disease prevention, strengthening self-care, health education, and comprehensive life planning.

There are several specific demographic and disease pattern changes that social work practice will need to address. Medical practice patterns have altered in response to changing clinical needs and shifts in financing. There are increases in the use, especially by the elderly patients, of sites other than the hospital for health care. Nursing home admissions increased sixty percent, community services have increased thirty-six percent and Medicare home health services by forty-seven percent in the past five years. The locations of health social work staffing and clinical activities have not shifted accordingly. Social work staff are not as available in these non-hospital sites as they have been in our acute facilities.

CHANGING HEALTH CARE NEEDS, EXTENDED LIFE EXPECTANCY AND INCREASING LEVELS OF DISABILITY

The movement to these new alternatives to hospital settings reflects a shift in the type of care needed as well as changing technological capabilities. The nation's health care system was designed for a younger, less ill population. The health care treatment paradigm is now shifting from acute to chronic care, especially with the growing proportion of elderly.

At the turn of the century Americans had an average life expectancy of approximately forty years. By 1992 it was nearly eighty years. While a significant factor in this change was the large decline in infant mortality, the size and proportion of the older population grew from four percent at the turn of the century to twelve percent in 1990. The oldest (75-100+) populations show dramatic expansion in both numbers and proportion of the total population. The eighty-five plus year-old population is the fastest growing segment of the population in the nation. Life expectancy at these older years has also dramatically expanded. Today a person who has already lived 100 years still has a life expectancy of 3.6 years.[4]

The incidence of illness and disability rises dramatically with advanced age, creating a need for considerable health care resources. Disability in these years due to physical or cognitive impairment can also result in loss of independence in activities of daily living such as bathing, dressing, continence, toileting independently and eating. Older adults make use of many health and personal care resources and therefore represent a large population for health care social work services. For example, this twelve percent of the United States' population uses:

- 1/3 of physician time
- Forty percent of hospital admissions
- Twenty-five percent of medications sold
- Thirty-six percent of personal health care expenditures.[5]

Presently, eighty percent of all deaths and ninety percent of all morbidity are the result of chronic disease; the vast majority of health care resources are focused on addressing the early detection and subsequent management of chronic care illnesses. Most health care costs occur at the end of a patient's life. Fifty percent of the average lifetime health expenditure occurs in the last two years of life and sixty percent of those expenditures occurs in the last six weeks of life.[6]

THE INTEGRATED CARE DELIVERY SYSTEM

Patients with chronic care needs, especially the elderly, will dominate the use of health care services and dollars in the decades ahead. The care needs of these individuals are enduring and not solely medical. It is likely that the patient will also require an array of supportive services such as meals, transportation, personal care, bathing, shopping and light housekeeping chores. Supervision, medication reminders, and assistance with transfer and toileting functions can also be crucial in keeping people with long-term needs out of the hospital and nursing home. Counseling to help people adapt to the need for supportive services and to ensure the appropriateness of the care plan is key to the successful care of chronic and disabling conditions. Respite care for involved family and friends is an additional critical feature. These services most frequently are provided in the home although they may be augmented by adult day care or may occur in assisted living settings. Intermittent or long-term use of nursing home/skilled nursing facility is a frequent component of care.

Social work skills in arranging complex community-based in-home services are valuable here. The historical strength of social work in patient advocacy, decision-making counseling, ethics committee work, facilitating patient self-determination and skills in helping families work to reach a consensus will have increasing value in the new health care delivery systems. Specifically, the following social work practice strengths are key in caring for this population.

1. Patient problems are multi-faceted and require services from a host of providers. Social work skill in complex care planning and service coordination is crucial.

2. The multiplicity of care providers addressing health and personal care are paid from a blend of public, private and out-of-pocket resources. Social work knowledge of payment regulation is very useful in coordinating care. Experience with a full array of income levels is relevant as well.

3. Families provide vast amounts of supportive care. Friends and neighbors provide other informal care. Social work skill in facilitating shared family decision-making and properly partialized caregiving is very useful. Family counseling skills are well used in this work.

4. Self-care is a critical element in managing chronic conditions to assure maintenance of maximum feasible health status. Social work health education and counseling skills are essential.

5. Mental competence, emotional and mental status are crucial factors in self-care. Social work skill in assessment, treatment and other related skills are valuable with this population.

6. Health social work experience in facilitating interdisciplinary care planning for ethically complex situations, and facilitating patient and family involvement in decision-making, is an important arena of professional expertise.

Health care coordination to identify specific needs and coordinate the plans from multiple providers into an integrated whole together with the physician is a natural social work role. This fact is being increasingly recognized by leading providers such as HMOs in their programs for seniors. An integrated delivery system is needed that melds biopsychosocial assessment and interventions, self-care regimens and coordination of complex medical in-home supportive services as an alternative to acute and skilled nursing facility care.

Social work is accustomed to focusing on the biopsychosocial interface, and has traditionally packaged services tied to brief medical care intervention to assure prudent use of high cost medical services. Health care social work in the current environment needs to provide strong conceptual leadership to pull the array of health care services together into coordinated, social work-directed community care management systems.

For the frail with persistent and complex care needs, social worker and nurses working as a team can provide physician-office and in-home assessments to assure appropriate and prudent deployment of needed complex personal care services. These services should not be limited to post-acute phases of care. Earlier intervention may prevent hospitalization and inappropriate use of Emergency Room. Short term rehabilitative/restorative services can help the patient regain the highest possible level of functioning which will also improve the quality of life and health status of the patient. This approach can also optimize the money available for patient care.

With older and disabled populations, the meaning of health promotion changes; the objective is to enhance the recovery process, to slow the deterioration occurring because of illness, and to retard the trend towards disability. It can include:

- prevention or delay of serious illness
- better management and diminished suffering from chronic conditions
- less frequent complications and reduced disability when disease develops
- comprehensive rehabilitation from serious illness.[7]

Specific supportive social work services need to be effectively located in key community care service providers: physician's offices, home health agencies, skilled nursing facilities as well as in residential settings and adult day care facilities. Case finding methods for short term interventions will need to be developed in each of these settings. Methods are also needed to identify patients with chronic conditions who need ongoing management and assistance.

AN EXAMPLE

Ambulatory Care/Social Work Outreach

Moving social work case finding into the primary care setting is a high priority within the perspective of integrated community-based chronic social/health care systems; especially as physicians are reemerging as the central clinical leaders. The internist/family practice office is an ideal new setting for social work. Over 85% of individuals in the 65 year-old and older category see a physician during each year. Social work services located in these settings allow early and comprehensive interventions to those in need, when they can have the most significant impact.

Models testing primary health care settings such as physician's office as access points to community care resources are emerging across the country under both social work and nursing leadership. One of the first such models was initiated in 1992 at Huntington Memorial Hospital under 30-month funding from John A. Hartford Foundation. This national project has additional sites at Baylor Hospital in Texas, Philadelphia Geriatric Center/Einstein Medical Center in Philadelphia and Beverly Hospital in Massachusetts. It is directed by Huntington Hospital's Senior Care Network, a comprehensive set of social work-led community-based care coordination programs. The project objectives of this hospital-physician partnership are to:

1. Develop criteria and methods to identify patients needing community care intervention.
2. Develop and test practical referral methods to assure physician and patient convenience in accessing new care resources.
3. Develop and test feedback systems to assure physician knowledge of community care.
4. Define, test and establish financing mechanisms for social work/care coordination services in the primary physician's office.

Although the Senior Care Network case management services had existed in the community for over eight years, physician use of these services was uneven and lacked consistent guidelines and criteria. It was anticipated that extending the social work role to the primary care setting would show the physician the value of social work services in medical care.

Having an immediate social work response system come to see the patient during the office visit turned out to be a central component. The benefits of the project were earlier social work intervention and thus prevention of patient decline, enhancement of restorative efforts and easy access to resources needed for improved patient compliance with prescribed medical care. Additional benefits were value-added marketing for physicians' practices to help to attract new patients and retain existing patients, reduction of liability risk through the addition of more comprehensive care especially for vulnerable and frail populations requiring care at home, and improved physician productivity. Payment sources are being tested. While the community-based case management program was originally considered the appropriate sponsor, experience suggests the hospital social work department or home health social work program are better first responders and therefore sponsors. The community case management program is the key solution for a significant portion but not the majority of patients, and thus becomes a receiving program.

COMMUNITY HEALTH FOCUS

Overall, the comprehensive community care focus is moving in the direction of payor-initiated efforts to enhance the health and functional status of chronically ill populations. The enhanced leadership role of physicians is central. The ability to target appropriate individuals for early intervention and enhance their ability to comply with needed self care regimens will slow their decline in health and diminish the need for the use of high cost health care resources such as emergency departments and inpatient hospital care. This approach should enhance quality of patients' lives while reducing the total cost of health care across the population. These strategies make sense under any system, but have particular efficacy within capitated managed care systems in which both physician and hospital are at financial risk, and have incentives to optimize health status across populations.[8]

Under these financial incentives, new opportunities emerge. For instance, the definition of the insurance-based case manager can be broadened dramatically to incorporate the capabilities of social work-directed community care services to optimize patient health and reduce disability status over time.

People with the same chronic illness may have various functional differences. These differential outcomes are frequently tied to basic lifestyle issues:

- proper nutrition
- smoking
- alcohol abuse
- adequate social involvement
- physical activity/exercise
- management of multiple medications
- availability of social support.

Interventions that optimize patient self-care and family supportive management include:

- Education of patient and family to basic lifestyle and compliance issues and their consequences for medical management;
- Counseling and encouragement to motivate patients to apply their understanding of these lifestyle factors to their own self management;
- Consultation to help patients and families understand how to access and use appropriate resources to facilitate self management;
- Guidance through the maze of service resources to pay for needed care;
- Assistance in mobilizing natural resources such as families and neighbors;
- Counseling to encourage adherence to agreed-on care plans and working through barriers to them.

CONCLUSION

These are times of needed fundamental system redesign in the delivery of both health care and the community care systems necessary to help manage patients with chronic conditions. In addition to a comprehensive continuum of care, coordinating mechanisms are needed to ensure the proper management of complex/high medical and personal care resource-utilizing patient populations. Early intervention through prevention, health education, life planning, insurance counseling and health promotion education will be important strategies. Development and refinement of criteria to precisely identify patients who need additional social work services in order to maintain optimum health at appropriate costs are vital new directions. As the primary care setting is where the greatest majority of patients are seen and early detection can most readily occur, it is the most critical arena for social work health care service delivery redesign. This strategic approach to health care should occur in close partnership with overall health care redesign and be attached to shifting patterns of health care funding. This approach will assure the centrality of social work/community care resources to support these important new methods for addressing patients with chronic illness or who are at the end stage of their lives.

NOTES

1. Goldsmith, Jeff. "The Paradigm Shift." *Decisions in Imaging Economics.* 1990.
2. Health One Corporation. *The Trauma of Transformation in the 1990's.* 1989.
3. American Hospital Association. "Ambulatory Surgery." *Ambulatory Care Trend Lines.* Vol. I, #2. 1992. Chicago, IL.
4. Society of Actuaries. *Group Annuity Mortality Table.* 1983.
5. Health One Corporation. *The Trauma of Transformation in the 1990's.* 1989.
6. Lubitz, J., Prihoda, R. "Use and Cost of Medicare Services in the Last Two Years of Life." *Health Care Financing Review* 5:117-31. 1984.
7. Levin, Robert C., Maloney, Susan K. *An Employer's Guide to Health Promotion for Older Workers & Retirees.* Washington Business Group on Health. Institute on Aging, Work & Health. 1993.
8. White, M., Simmons, W.J., Bixby, N. "Managed Care and Case Management: An Overview." *Discharge Planning Update.* Volume 13, #1. January-February 1993.

REFERENCES

American Hospital Association. (1992). "Ambulatory surgery." *Ambulatory Care Trend Lines.* Volume I, #2.
Goldsmith, Jeff. (1990). "The paradigm shift." *Decisions in Imaging Economics.*
Health One Corporation. (1989). *The Trauma of Transformation in the 1990's.*

Levin, Robert C., Maloney, Susan K. (1993). *An Employer's Guide to Health Promotion for Older Workers & Retirees.* Washington Business Group on Health. Institute on Aging, Work & Health.

Lubitz, J., Prihoda, R. (1984). "Use and cost of medicare services in the last two years of life." *Health Care Financing Review* 5:117-31.

Society of Actuaries. (1983). *Group Annuity Mortality Table.*

U.S. Select Committee on Aging. (1991). *Aging America: Trends and Projections.*

White, M., Simmons, W.J., Bixby, N. (January-February 1993). "Managed care and case management: An overview." *Discharge Planning Update.* Volume 13, #1.

PART 3:
ARTICLES

Managed Care and Social Work: Constructing a Context and a Response

Donald S. Cornelius, MSW

SUMMARY. Managed care is described as a strategy developed by the health care industry as a means to control profitability in the dispersement of health care resources. Control of utilization, cost and information are the essential elements of this strategy. The potential impact of each strategy on social work practice is explored. A number of suggestions are made to insure that managed care balances the needs of its corporate sponsors with those of the consumer public and providers of health care.

AN EXPLANATION OF MANAGED CARE

Managed care is a collective term that is being used to represent a host of different, sometimes conflicting, ideas about health care

Donald S. Cornelius is Director of Research and Program Development with the Behavioral Counseling Associates of Long Island.

[Haworth co-indexing entry note]: "Managed Care and Social Work: Constructing a Context and a Response." Cornelius, Donald S. Co-published simultaneously in *Social Work in Health Care* (The Haworth Press, Inc.) Vol. 20, No. 1, 1994, pp. 47-63; and: *Social Work in Ambulatory Care: New Implications for Health and Social Services* (ed: Gary Rosenberg, and Andrew Weissman) The Haworth Press, Inc., 1994, pp. 47-63. Multiple copies of this article/chapter may be purchased from The Haworth Document Delivery Center [1-800-3-HAWORTH; 9:00 a.m. - 5:00 p.m. (EST)].

delivery and resource management. Most often it is presented as a management strategy to contain the escalation of health care costs. In managed care, a case manager is a third party in the dispensation of medical services. Physicians and other health care providers must have the type and quantity of care approved by the case manager prior to, or closely associated with, the giving of care. Managed care is also used to represent strategies to insure more adequate health care for the poor and disadvantaged, as a way to insure quality health care by the closer scrutiny of care providers and users, or as a potential technique to shift the emphasis in health care away from the management of acute and chronic illness toward a concern for prevention. It is not unusual to find these notions woven together into arguments that justify the necessity of managing the freedom of providers and the recipients of health care to utilize the finite resources available for health concerns.

A discussion of managed care could easily become a debate about whether and to what extent managed care fulfills its intended goals. For example, Daniel Borenstein (1990) sees managed care as a rationing of care that ultimately deprives patients of quality care. Daniel Patterson (1990), in the same publication, portrays managed care as an approach to the rational treatment of psychiatric patients and therefore an insurer of quality treatment. Another debated issue is the question of cost containment. Despite cost control being touted as the primary goal of managed care, it is not at all clear that managed care will be able to accomplish this intention. Donald Moran and Patricia Wolfe (1991) present managed care as an untested strategy that may or may not be able to contain the escalation of cost. As yet there is promise but questionable evidence (Schwartz and Mendelson, 1992). It is not the purpose of this paper to engage in the debate about the adequacy or inadequacy of managed care to fulfill its publicized mission, but to search out its place in the development of the current health care environment and to speculate about what meaning it may have for social workers.

A CONTEXT FOR MANAGED CARE

In its essence managed care is a strategy for the control of how health care dollars are spent. Victor Fuchs (1986), a health care economist, argues that the current awareness that the public and private sector cannot devote unlimited financial resources to health care has caused a "battle for control" (p. 300) among the various health care interests: provider physicians, other health care professionals and their facilities, the corporate health care industry and government. Managed care is only the latest effort on the part of government, and more aggressively, the health insurance industry, to attain dominance in this battle. The stakes are high for everyone. Providers wish to protect their sources of income; industry and government are under pressure to contain health care expenditures; and the medical industry wishes to protect and increase its profitability. It is important to note that the health care consumer is conspicuously absent from this array.

The battle, while drawn, is not among equals any one of whom might emerge as the victor. Quite the contrary, the use of managed care is a signal that, while skirmishes may continue, the outcome is already determined by the managers. The basis for this conclusion rests on several factors. First is the marked expansion in the last twenty years of health and welfare corporations. According to Paul Starr (1982) and Davis Stoesz (1986), the private corporate sector has been steadily assuming control of human services that were traditionally in the hands of voluntary and public agencies. Stoesz calls this development "corporate welfare."

The Health Maintenance Act of 1973 encouraged private proprietary firms to develop and market health care for profit. As these corporations developed they made loans and stock offerings with the understanding that profits were to be made for investors. Discovering the potential for financial gain by providing welfare services, corporations built hospitals, nursing homes, home care firms, and health maintenance organizations as profit-making opportunities. As privately held businesses they were and continue to be somewhat free of regulations and can exercise an unencumbered hand in establishing practices promoting business profitability as a priority. Managed care is one such practice that is meant to represent the interests of the health care industry in controlling costs, and more importantly, in allocating resources. Only when the health care industry controls these elements can it insure itself and its investors a profit.

A second factor in understanding the context for managed care is the extent to which business and industry, both as payer and provider, now control the field. Betty Leyerle (1984) notes that from the 1970s to the present there has been a steady drift away from the professional to the bureaucratic control of health care. In this transition she sees a shift in focus away from service, the essence of professionalism, toward meeting the goals of organizations, the essence of bureaucratization. While health care is a service industry, all industry by its nature put corporate viability above the consumers of its products. Business needs to control the means and resources required for product production so as to protect its stake in its industry. This is no less true in the business of health care. To understand the place of managed care in the current health care environment, particularly for social work, a review of how managerial control has developed is in order.

CONTROL OF UTILIZATION

Leyerle (1984) describes three areas where the health care industry has moved gradually to achieve dominance: controlling the utilization of health care, controlling payment for care, and the control of information. The control of utilization is achieved primarily through control of the providers. Thus, physician's services were the first target. The health industry rode on the coattails of the federal government's attempts to contain the cost of Medicare. In 1967, Congress made Medicare providers demonstrate that utilized care was necessary and reasonable. This first effort at containment seemed to have no effect on cost reduction. To strengthen utilization review (UR) the 1972 Congress created the peer standards review organization (PSRO). Selected billings were to be reviewed by medical peers to insure and certify proper utilization of services. Improper utilization potentially meant loss of payment. Since peer review was less than effective, the next step in the control of utilization was diagnostic related groups (DRGs). In 1983 state and local governments, then the federal government, began forcing hospitals and physicians to plan care before rendering services based upon the patient's diagnosis. Through these mechanisms the health care professions became acclimated, though grudgingly, to the justification of their professional decisions and the way care was managed.

Gradually, the application of UR, PR and DRGs was extended to the private sector as the corporate payers of employee benefits also sought to contain the escalation of medical costs. Through these review procedures, those who were paying for the service had a means to monitor how and what services were rendered. Control of care and medical service was no longer a monopoly of the providers, the physicians. These review procedures established an important precedent that has become a basic assumption of the current health care culture, namely, health care providers must be watched and controlled (Leyerle, 1984).

Managed care extends the watchful eye of utilization review into primary care, as well. Until the advent of managed care most utilization control measures were limited to services rendered in hospitals, nursing homes and other secondary care facilities. Primary care for the most part remained free of such scrutiny. Managed care is an important new strategy because it exposes every type of service offered in any setting by any health care provider to the review of the case manager. Undermanaged care utilization is firmly in the hands of that part of the health care industry that is in control of funding. What is particularly fascinating about this development is that cost control through control of utilization is now an almost uncontested right of the managers who handle the purse.

As a result of these shifts in accountability the social worker becomes directly involved in the control of utilization, either as an agency employee or as a private practitioner. Managed care only succeeds if the routine practice of the provider is monitored carefully. Therefore, every client's case must be structured according to the protocols of the managed care firm. To insure accountability, managed care agencies require direct contact with the person providing the service. For this reason many managed care providers will not certify agencies but only individual providers whom they have determined to be qualified. This is a powerful tool in the hands of the managed care entity because the social worker then serves only at their discretion. Licensing and credentials, governmental and professional, are not sufficient to qualify. The provider requires the additional certification of the managed care entity.

This presents some significant difficulties for social workers in servicing their clients. By participating in managed care the social worker's practice becomes bound by the contract made with the managed care company before the client is seen or assessed. In essence, the social worker becomes an agent of managed care and agrees to serve the public within the corporate guidelines and not necessarily according to the assessed needs of the client. The status of the social worker as agent is enforced by the power to give or withhold reimbursement for the services rendered. If the social worker practices outside the protocols, the case manager has the power to deny payment. The client is denied coverage and the social worker is denied reimbursement; money becomes both carrot and stick.

CONTROL OF COST

Control of utilization is reinforced through control of the financial resources allocated to health care, the second area to be considered. Almost all health care dollars originate from two sources, employee benefits and the three levels of government. After World War II the notion that health insurance was a right of employment became firmly established. Medicare and Medicaid conveyed the same rights to the old, the poor, the disabled and unemployable. A huge and reliable source of money was now available to pay for health services that initially had few restrictions on its use. The health insurance industry was given the job of managing these resources. But this has also changed the nature of the insurance industry from managing risk to managing money. There is little insurance risk in health care at present. Insurance companies act as agents of government and the private sector monitoring and distributing health care dollars. A primary source of income for these companies is derived from fees charged to manage health care expenditures.

These services are called "products" by the insurance industry. Products represent different strategies of management and the policies the managers will use in distributing each buyer's health care dollars. The possibilities are unlimited and can incorporate any requirements as long as the buyer of the product is willing to pay.

The insurance industry tailors a product to meet the current needs of the marketplace and the agenda of the moment. At present, cost control is the pressing issue and insurance companies are selling products which promise cost containment.

Managed care, itself, is such a cost containment product. The insurance industry is selling a promise to limit cost increases and a means to do so which is termed 'managing care.' Claims for reimbursement submitted through managed care are paid out only when they meet the criteria for care preset by the buyer of the health care package and the managed care company. These criteria, called protocols, are said to meet the community standards for medical care. However, they also contain the benefit limits the buyer of the managed care product wishes to provide. In managing the care, the case manager determines both whether the service is medically necessary and if it is a service covered by the commercial contract. Practicing this way increases the potential of confusing managerial necessity with medical necessity. It is important to emphasize that these standards are not used capriciously or without regard to medical concerns. The point here is one of control. Managed care puts the balance of control into the hands of the insurance companies that are promising cost containment to satisfy the buyers of their products. Managed care has other items in its agenda, but cost control is its main reason for being (Coopers & Lybrand, 1991; Gary, 1991).

Managed care has extended the cost containment strategy to social work provider as well. Fee negotiation and payment agreements are no longer between the social worker and the client. Fee arrangements have been determined by the managed care contract. The client usually pays nothing or a small co-payment to the provider. The primary billing and fee collection are between the managed care company and the social worker. Such an arrangement solidifies the perception of all concerned that the provider social worker is an agent of managed care.

Another control strategy using the financial carrot and stick is discounting. Managed care personnel suggest that by lowering the fee and by controlling utilization the social worker will be designated the preferred provider in their area. The social worker agrees contractually with the managed care firm to provide service for a fee lower than the one which might be standard in a locality. An increase in referrals is implied, but never promised as an incentive to lower the fee. Meanwhile the social worker has lost control of pricing services. Any future fee changes will have to be negotiated through the managed care company. Thus managed care decreases the scope and flexibility of the social worker's professional autonomy through controlling the disbursement of economic resources and the utilization of services.

CONTROL OF INFORMATION

Information control is the third area of dominance which brings perspective to our understanding of managed care. Leyerle (1986) observes that the systems of control are only possible through the control of data and statistics all of which are in the hands of the insurance companies. The imposition of DRGs and peer review established the concept that it is possible to lay out a course of treatment and a level of care for any one illness. It has become the practice when evaluating care to use these established patterns as the standards against which current treatments are to be judged. These standards have been codified within the insurance industry and form the basis for treatment protocols.

Over the last twenty years insurance companies have been collecting information about the utilization of treatment. On the surface this approach seems reasonable, if it were not for several factors which raise questions about its reliability. First, the insurance companies generally consider this information privileged and part of their confidential business practices. Insurance companies do not generally tell providers and patients the content of their standards when treatment is being certified or when a claim is being evaluated. While the data is based upon information given by the provider about the patient's treatment, neither can gain access to it or the ways it is used. This raises questions about medical information as a privileged communication between provider and patient.

The second problem with standards is that insurance companies control the protocols by the kinds of information they collect and through the application of the standard itself. For example, many managed care products now specify that short term psychotherapy is the appropriate level of care for marital problems. Consequently, the case manager will only certify short term counseling as the appropriate level of care for marital dysfunction. Provider and client must operate under this protocol to receive reimbursement. When treatment statistics are subsequently collected, they will show that short term therapy was the type of treatment most often used and will become an important part of establishing that the appropriate standard of care for marital problems is short term therapy. Is short term therapy the most effective treatment or the most efficient, that is, cost effective? It could be one or the other or both, but how are we to know?

Control of information is a powerful tool used to define the way in which health care is dispensed. Once again the balance of power is clearly in the hands of the insurance industry. The industry justifies this by the need to keep business practices confidential and by the fact that physicians, nurses, social workers, and other professional health care personnel are on the inside managing these programs. There is the implication that even within the corporate world, health care professionals will be guided by their professional ethics. It remains to be seen what comfort can be taken by these reassurances. As the insurance industry markets its managed care products, how can we evaluate its promise of containing costs and improving the quality of care unless there is access to information?

The control of information solidifies the control of social work services under managed care. Standards of care and the protocols which guide them can only be exercised through the disclosure of information. The social worker becomes both the collector of information about the client and the conduit of that data to the managed care case manager. Analysis of the diagnosis and functional impairment of the client is measured against the protocols in establishing eligibility for service. Once given, the social worker has little control of the analysis or the use of the information.

As an illustration of this process we can return to the earlier example of marital dysfunction. A particular managed care contract may allow or disallow care for such a presenting problem. The determination of reimbursement is not based upon the functional impairment such a problem represents for the client but upon whether it is covered in the commercial contract establishing the managed care agreement. Another example, though extreme, can be cited which illustrates how clearly business priorities can prevail over medical need. In 1990 several firms in Texas sought to disallow any coverage for AIDS care whether or not it related to medical necessity. The insurance companies representing those firms were willing and able to write AIDS patients out of their contractual arrangement.

Social workers providing information have no way of knowing whether the information will be used for their clients' good or ill. It is important to stress that managed care products have no consistent set of inclusions. Their variation is truly infinite. Yet full disclosure is required as a condition for determining the client's eligibility for reimbursement. These examples are not meant to imply that managed care is merely looking for ways to avoid liability, but rather, to emphasize the way in which information provided by the social worker is used for purposes determined by the managed care firm and those who engage them. The interests of the social worker's client are made secondary by the process itself.

Managed care is being promoted as the best possible answer to the containment of health care costs. Whether managed care will be any more successful at this effort than past attempts remains to be seen. However, according to this analysis of managed care, cost containment will be a secondary gain. It is more instructive to see managed care as one more incremental step in placing health care under corporate dominance. The mechanisms to establish and maintain these controls are now well in place: utilization and peer review, diagnostic related groups, standards of care and most recently, managed care.

Leaders of the insurance industry naturally maintain this is a positive development and an opportunity to bring a comprehensive planning to the provision of health care. They see themselves as perfectly positioned, a position they have consciously constructed, to be the axis of control for the management of the many diverse issues related to the current and future provision of health care. James Lynn (1991), the chairman of Aetna Life and Casualty, portrays his industry as the one social institution possessing the comprehensive expertise that will insure both the efficient and effective provision of health care. The business community, however, is not a benign entity in this process.

CONSTRUCTING A SOCIAL WORK RESPONSE
TO MANAGED CARE

The role of the social worker is rapidly changing as a result of the development of corporate welfare. Traditionally, social work has functioned as part of the voluntary sector. As a result, the field of social work has not been in a position to greatly impact the corporate world. Yet recent shifts have put social work into the midst of the managed care stream. Social workers are finding themselves providing social work services inside the hospitals, nursing homes, home care agencies and many other health related institutions that are organized as profit making businesses (Poole and Braja, 1984; Robinson, 1989; Edinburg and Cottler, 1990; Midanik, 1991). Managed care has proven to be a boon for job opportunities for social workers as corporate insiders: social workers function in the capacity of case managers, supervisors of case managers, systems auditors, policy analysts, and even as the developers and sales people of managed care products (Bickerton, 1990; Wagman and Schiff, 1990). An additional factor in this change has been the growing number of social workers in independent practice who have joined the ranks of those in the business of health care (Kurzman, 1976; Alexander, 1987; Barker, 1991; Matorin et al., 1987; Courtney, 1992).

Managed care as a corporate strategy to control the utilization of health care for profit is an important perspective in constructing a response to managed care. It is important to remember that over the last thirty years the monopoly in health care has changed hands from the providers, the physicians, to the corporate boards and managers. This battle of the titans, as Fuchs (1986) notes, continues. As a possible response, social workers might be tempted to join one side or the other, whichever are more sympathetic to the interests of social work. The resulting dominance of either providers or the health care industry can only serve to maintain the interests of one side or the other at public expense. A more meaningful response would be to find ways to dilute the monopolies that have been operative in health care.

It is essential for the profession to encourage legislation that imposes some regulation on managed care. Currently there are almost no state or federal laws which regulate managed care companies' policies and procedures. The climate for such controls is emerging. In 1981, 290 billion dollars was spent on health care; in 1991, 738 billion (Pear, 1992). This cost escalation has fostered a change in the political climate toward a reexamination of the place of regulation in determining health care goals and policy. Disillusionment with deregulation and the encouragement of the free market in health care, the principal cost containment strategies of the Reagan administration, has led the way for regulatory intervention. Government is the only institution large and powerful enough to make a meaningful change. State legislatures are again becoming active in imposing planning and controls on how the health care industry operates under their jurisdictions (Pear, 1992). In such an environment, legislation regulating the rules under which managed care operates might be seen as one component of the effort to dilute corporate dominance of the field. Legislation might insure that the public has access to all health care providers, for example.

Managed care firms should not be able to require additional certification and limit access to providers who have already been licensed by the states to provide health care. This corporate and non-regulated certification is the key to managed care's achievement of dominance over providers. Corporate certification limits access of consumers solely to their approved agents. Furthermore, it gives managed care firms the ability to screen providers not only on their competence in rendering care but on the extent to which they comply with case management. A restive provider who may disagree with a case manager can easily be decertified with no legally sanctioned recourse or knowledge of the terms of his/her changed status.

Another growing example of corporate dominance that might be regulated is the control of information. There is no justification for managed care firms to maintain that protocols determining care are trade secrets. If clients must open their confidential conversations with their providers to access care, then managed care firms must be forced to reciprocate. Lack of public access to information about managed care will allow corporations to construct the management of health care on terms consistent with their goals and interests without public debate. How will the public know whether the standards being established by managed care operate to improve the efficiency and effectiveness of health care? Furthermore, providers should be aware of the ways in which the information they provide and the care they are permitted to render are constructing the future of their professional conduct.

In a similar fashion social workers can dilute corporate agenda setting by taking responsibility for the research and analysis of the data which their practice generates. This approach could potentially promote and advocate for social work's particular perspective on health and wellness. There is much literature concerning social work research as a means of validating and confirming the efficacy of social work practice. At times this research agenda may be structured to justify social work as a valid form of intervention to the current health care establishment (McCuan et al., 1991). While this is certainly one possible goal for the social work research agenda, the profession needs to conduct research and advocate for its particular perspective on health care as an end in itself (Monkman, 1991).

Another means to influence the managed care system involves joining with other health care professionals in asserting their essential role in the provision of health care and the value base which traditionally defines these professions. Managed care will not succeed without the cooperation of the provider community. Corporate managed care must be made aware that social workers have a dual stake in their response: advocacy for client services and the maintenance of the profession for this task. The integrity of the social work profession is maintained only when clients' needs and the advocacy for those needs are its first concern.

A further strategy for gaining influence is for social workers to use every contact with case managers to express their priority, that is, meeting the needs of the client. While professional organizations are beginning to take an active role in this assertion, there is a more immediate way to make a point-of-service impression. Managed care is still in its infancy in its attempts to micro manage the delivery of care. Now is the time for providers to assert their professional perspective on the treatments allowed and the allocation of treatment while there is still incentive to modify and reevaluate initial protocols.

Finally, a social work response to managed care should involve caution in defining its practice narrowly within a medical framework. Managed care is currently being framed as a means to manage medical costs, and this is defined as managing the utilization of medical technology. In seeking the reimbursement of many of its services under mental health care, the field of social work has left itself vulnerable to having its services defined as merely medical-like interventions and therefore evaluated as either medically unnecessary or non-efficacious from a medical perspective.

It is important to recognize that managed care can be one possible legitimate and necessary strategy to manage the cost and utilization of health care. It may also achieve the goal of a more equitable distribution of health care resources. There is much about the stated intent of managed care that social workers may wish to support: (1) the control of the utilization of health care resources for treatments that are efficacious and necessary, (2) the need to control the proportion of private and public resources spent on health care at the expense of other social needs and problems, (3) the utilization of public money to improve and maintain the health of the poor and disabled rather than an emphasis on treatment of illness alone, (4) the opportunity to educate the public about the proportionate use of health care services and the distinction between medical need and personal want. The dilemma for the profession is how to insure that managed care begins to serve these ends rather than the ends of corporate control.

A SOCIAL WORK VALUE ORIENTATION

Managed care is a potential quagmire for social work either as provider or as corporate insider. As the profession seeks to construct and advocate for its own definitions of health and wellness, maintenance of its values and ethical standards will provide perspective in these entanglements. In the conclusion of his book, *Who Shall Live,* Victor Fuchs (1975) observes that most contemporary health problems and concerns are rarely a matter of the application of medical technology and care:

> At the root of most of our major health problems are value choices: What kind of people are we? What kind of life do we want to lead? What kind of society do we want to build for our children and grandchildren? How much weight do we want to give to individual freedom? how much to equality? how much to material progress? how much to the realm of the spirit? How important is our own health to us? How important is our neighbors' health to us? The answers we give to these questions will and should shape health care policy. (p. 148)

Thus managed care cannot be approached from a narrow focus as if it were just one more wrinkle in the evolving structure of medical care in the United States to which social work and other health care providers will make accommodations. This may in fact happen. However, if this is the only response social work makes to managed care it will have failed to raise the value questions that are inherent in the way managed care is presently structured. An opportunity and a responsibility exists for the field of social work to influence the character and organization of managed care (Dane and Simon, 1991).

Charles Levy (1984) notes that one of the essential cultural functions of social work is the provision of human services from the value perspective embodied in the NASW Code of Ethics. Social work as a socially constructed institution is meant to use these standards to define its practice conduct and to craft its social policies and social actions. The primacy of the client and the maintenance of a just and equitable social order are the foundation of these ethical principles. Social work has much to say to and about managed care and must take this charge seriously.

REFERENCES

Alexander, M.P. (1987). Why social workers enter private practice: A study of motivation and attitudes. *Journal of Independent Social Work, 1*, (3), 7-18.

Barker, R.L. (1991). *Social work in private practice.* Washington D.C.: NASW Press.

Bickerton, R.L. (1990). Employee assistance: A history in progress. *EAP Digest, 11,* (1), 34.

Borenstein, D.B. (1990). Managed care: A means of rationalizing psychiatric treatment. *Hospital and Community Psychiatry, 41,* (10), 1095-98.

Coopers & Lybrand. (1991). *The managed care industry-1991* (Industrial Profile Series). New York: Author.

Courtney, M. (1992). Psychiatric social work and the early days of private practice. *Social Service Review, 66,* (2), 199-214.

Dane, B.O., Simon, B.L. (1991). Resident guests: Social workers in host settings. *Social Work, 36,* (3), 208-213.

Edinburg, G., Cottler, J. (1990). Implications of managed care for social work in psychiatric hospitals. *Hospital and Community Psychiatry, 41,* (10), 1063-64.

Fuchs, V. (1975). *Who shall live? Health, economics and social choice.* New York: Basic Books.

Fuchs, V. (1986). *The health economy.* Cambridge: Harvard University Press.

Gary, W.B. (1991). *Implementing managed health care* (Report Number 968). Washington D.C.: The Conference Board.

Kurzman, P. (1976). Private practice as a social work function. *Social Work, 21,* (5), 363-368.

Levy, C. (1984). Values and ethics: Foundations for social work. In S. Dillick, (Ed.), *Value foundations of social work: Ethical basis for a human service profession.* Detroit: School of Social Work, Wayne State University.

Leyerle, B. (1984). *Moving and shaking medicine: The structure of a socioeconomic transformation.* Westport: Greenwood Press.

Lynn, J.T. (1991). Promise of managed care: An insurer's perspective. *Health Affairs, 10,* (4), 185-188.

Matorin, S., Rosenberg, B., Levitt, M., Rosenbaum, S. (1987). Private practice in social work: Readiness and opportunity. *Social Casework, 68,* (1), 31-37.

McCuan, E.R., Harbert, T.L., Fulton, J.R. (1991). Evaluation as imperative for social services preservation: A challenge to the Department of Veteran Affairs. *Journal of Social Work Education, 27,* (2), 114-124.

Midanik, L.T. (1991). Employee assistance programs: Lessons from history. *Employee Assistance Quarterly, 6,* (4), 69-77.

Monkman, M.M. (1991). Outcome objectives in social work practice: Person and environment. *Social Work, 36,* (3), 253-258.

Moran, D., Wolfe, P. (1991). Can managed care control costs? *Health Affairs, 10,* (4), 120-128.

Patterson, D.Y. (1990). Managed care: An approach to rational psychiatric treatment. *Hospital and Community Psychiatry, 41,* (10), 1092-95.

Pear, R. (1992, May 11). States are moving to reregulation on health costs. *New York Times,* A-1 & 10.

Poole, D.L., Braja, L.J. (1984). Does social work in HMOs measure up to professional standards? *Health and Social Work, 9,* (4), 305-313.

Robinson, M.O. (1989). Relationships between HMOs and mental health providers. *Social Casework, 70,* (10), 195-200.

Schwartz, W.B., Mendelson, D.N. (1992). Why managed care cannot contain hospital costs. *Health Affairs, 11*, (2), 100-107.

Starr, P. (1982). *The social transformation of american medicine.* New York: Basic Books.

Stoesz, D. (1986). Corporate welfare: The third stage of welfare in the United States. *Social Work, 31*, (4), 245-249.

Wagman, J.B., Schiff, J. (1989). Managed mental health care for employees: Roles for social work. *Employee Assistance Quarterly, 6*, (3), 1-12.

Impact of Social Work on Recidivism and Non-Medical Complaints in the Emergency Department

Debra S. Keehn, MSW
Cathy Roglitz, ACSW
M. Leora Bowden, ACSW

SUMMARY. Recidivism among patients treated in the hospital Emergency Department (ED) is a significant factor in resource depletion. This study substantiates the efficacy of social work intervention in the ED using recidivism as an outcome measure. Data was collected on all patients seen by social work during the first 12 months of social work services to the ED between the hours of 3:00 p.m. and 11:30 p.m. The greatest decline in recidivism occurred where social work used a proactive intervention strategy as opposed to a more support oriented intervention.

INTRODUCTION

Recidivism and non-medical complaints among patients treated in the hospital emergency department (ED) are significant factors in

Debra Keehn is Clinical Social Worker, Cathy Roglitz is Social Work Specialist, and M. Leora Bowden is Senior Social Worker, Department of Social Work, University of Michigan Medical Center, 1500 E. Medical Center Drive, Ann Arbor, MI 48109.

[Haworth co-indexing entry note]: "Impact of Social Work on Recidivism and Non-Medical Complaints in the Emergency Department." Keehn, Debra S., Cathy Roglitz, and M. Leora Bowden. Co-published simultaneously in *Social Work in Health Care* (The Haworth Press, Inc.) Vol. 20, No. 1, 1994, pp. 65-75; and: *Social Work in Ambulatory Care: New Implications for Health and Social Services* (ed: Gary Rosenberg, and Andrew Weissman) The Haworth Press, Inc., 1994, pp. 65-75. Multiple copies of this article/chapter may be purchased from The Haworth Document Delivery Center [1-800-3-HAWORTH; 9:00 a.m. - 5:00 p.m. (EST)].

resource depletion. These problems drain the insurance industry, the medical centers, and the medical personnel who care for these patients. In the United States alone, patients with non-medical complaints absorb roughly 20% of all health care expenditures (Corr, 1992). Comparative studies on recidivists remain undocumented, as does the extent to which these two issues overlap. With the cost of medical care exploding and access to it becoming more difficult, cost containment thus becomes paramount to the health care industry.

Numerous authors (Bennett, 1973; Strinsky, 1970; Silverman, 1986; Moonilal, 1982; Lindenberg, 1972) have described the role of social work in the ED. However, it has only been in the past year that authors have attempted to document the impact of social work on the ED. Ponto and Berg (1992) assessed the cost benefit of a social work service in the ED, and Boyack and Bucknum (1992) documented that the presence of a social worker in the ED led to a reduction of non-acute admissions. The present study extends previous discussions by illustrating how social work can enhance patient care and interrupt cycles that deplete resources and impede service delivery in the ED medical system. This study substantiates the efficacy of social work intervention in the ED of a major midwest trauma center using recidivism as an outcome measure.

While efficient and accurate medical assessment is the crucial function of any ED, failure to address psychosocial components can produce costly consequences as incomplete assessment and discharge planning perpetuate recidivism. Because medical personnel rarely have the time and training to address the psychosocial basis of non-medical complaints and recidivism in the ED, and because medical personnel are seldom aware of community resources, social workers become invaluable team members who can identify issues related to problematic help-seeking behavior. Likewise, varying perceptions exist across the medical disciplines with respect to patients who could benefit from social work intervention (Dove, Schneider, & Gitelson, 1985). Thus, social work in the ED is a way to manage the costly problem of recidivists who present non-medical complaints, illustrating that patient care costs can be effectively contained, and that care itself can be enhanced by consistent identification of those in need of social work attention.

It has only been in recent years that medical social workers have encountered pressure to quantify the outcome of their interventions. With increased competition for funding and institutional down-sizing, social workers are now expected to measure the impact of their efforts. When compared to other professions, though, there remains a paucity of empirical studies by medical social workers, and none to date that substantiates social work on the basis of outcome studies with ED patients. This study demonstrates that social workers can have a positive influence on the problems of non-medical complaints and recidivism in the ED.

METHODS AND MATERIALS

The study was conducted in the ED at University of Michigan Medical Center (UMMC). The Medical Center is an 888 bed tertiary care hospital with an ED that has an average of 40,000 patient visits per year. Data were collected on 1,758 ED patients seen by social work between the hours of 3 p.m. and 11:30 p.m. during this 12 month study. This coincided with the introduction of social work services to the ED. Patients were referred to social work by ED personnel, or they were identified by social work based on stated complaints and general presentation. The two social workers assigned to provide services completed a survey after each intervention. There was no missing data, and uncertainty about patient information was clarified from lab test results, and from hospital records. Variables included referral source to social work, time spent by the social worker, insurance, gender, age, marital status, service provided by the social worker, disposition of patient, substance abuse, child/adult abuse, referral provided by the social worker, diagnosis, and recidivism. The variable Diagnosis was comprised of two categories, "Medical" (i.e., medical evaluation revealed a problem in need of treatment) and "Non-Medical" (i.e., medical evaluation revealed no problem in need of medical treatment).

Seven interventions were employed by social work: (1) crisis intervention; (2) patient support; (3) psychosocial assessment; (4) discharge planning; (5) tangible service; (6) family support; and (7) consultation to medical staff. Interventions were either support oriented (i.e., tangible services, patient support, family support) or proactive (e.g., crisis intervention, discharge planning, psychosocial assessment, consultation). Recidivism was operationally defined as presenting to the ED at least once 3 months preceding the initial social work intervention, or at least once 3 months post-intervention with social work. Recidivist data were included on their first presentation only. One methodological shortcoming of the study is that patients who ceased to be recidivists at UMMC could have gone to other facilities. However, many of the non-medical recidivists had restricted mobility as a result of homelessness and lack of transportation, in addition to significant histories with UMMC. Nevertheless, more research is needed on the recidivist population, and tracking medical involvements with related life events would be a contribution to the literature. A significance level of .01 was set for all comparisons. Figure 1 presents the flow chart followed by patients receiving social work intervention in the ED.

RESULTS

This heterogenous sample was 53% (n = 936) female, and 47% (n = 822) male. Age was standardized into years, with an overall average of 40 (min = 1; max = 98). Marital status distributions indicated that 52% (n = 909) were single, 30% (n = 534) married, 12% (n = 204) widowed, and 6% (n = 111) divorced. Patients with non-medical complaints represented 16% (n = 281) of the sample, those under the influence of alcohol 12% (n = 203), and those under the influence of other drugs roughly 4% (n = 73) of the sample. Disposition of ED patients following medical evaluation was as follows: 52% (n = 892) discharged, 46% (n = 774) admitted to the hospital, and 2% (n = 32) went to the morgue. With respect to arrival method, 56% (n = 958) arrived at the ED on their own, 32% (n = 549) by ambulance, 10% (n = 168) by helicopter, and 1% (n = 23) were brought in by local police.

Varying success rates as measured by recidivism were related to each respective intervention (see Figure 2). Because UMMC is a major trauma center, 24% (n = 418) of social work activity was family support. Patient support represented 32% (n = 559) of the interventions, psychosocial assessment 18% (n = 323), crisis intervention 12% (n = 209), discharge planning 10% (n = 178), consultation to medical staff 2% (n = 32), and 1% (n = 22, n = 17) each for grief

FIGURE 1

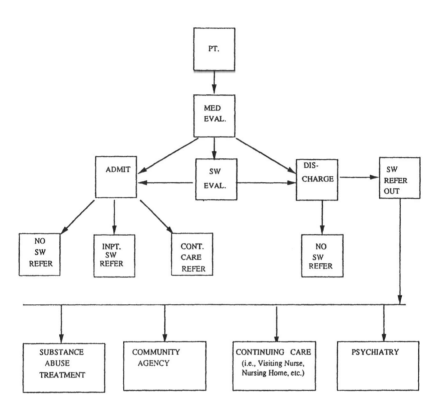

counseling, and tangible services. Recidivists three months prior to social work intervention accounted for 26.96% (n = 474) of the sample; recidivists three months after social work intervention accounted for 22.9% (n = 385) of the sample. A 4% (n = 89) decline in overall recidivism post-intervention is noteworthy given the wide range of costs possible for an ED visit. However, recidivism could be expected to decline most dramatically with the initial introduction of social work, and then to be managed over time with less dramatic changes due to early intervention designed to address the underlying precipitant for the ED visit.

Chi square tests for independence revealed respectable relationships: 42.3% (n = 119) of all pre-intervention patients with nonmedical complaints were recidivists (χ^2 = 40.2, df = 1, p < .01).

FIGURE 2. Recidivism by Service Pre- and Post-Intervention

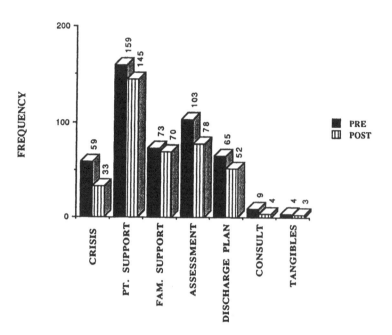

Three months post-intervention, however, this rate dropped to 27.7% (n = 78) (χ^2 = 6.7, df = 1, p < .01). See Figure 3.

Recidivism of alcohol abusers also declined from pre to post-intervention: 39.9% (n = 81) of all pre-intervention recidivists were legally intoxicated while only 23.1% (n = 47) of all post-intervention recidivists were intoxicated (χ^2 = 19.5, df = 1, p < .01). See Figure 4.

This result is attributed to the aggressive efforts of ED social work to triage these patients directly into substance abuse treatment from the ED. This patient population is especially relevant in terms of cost containment due to Michigan's Public Act 339, which mandates a medical treatment approach as opposed to incarceration. A full 51% (n = 891) of all patients seen by ED social work were given a referral including subsidized substance abuse treatment, Alcoholics Anonymous, Narcotics Anonymous, community mental health, homeless shelters, Department of Social Services, sexual assault programs, domestic violence programs, inpatient social

FIGURE 3. Recidivism by Diagnosis: Pre- and Post- Intervention

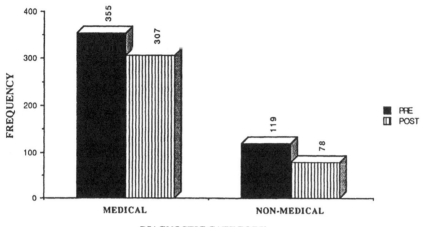

work for those admitted, and a variety of other specialized community-based resources. Overall, 55% (n = 111) of patients positive for alcohol did not require medical treatment though the remaining 45% (n = 92) were in need of immediate medical attention as a result of motor vehicle accidents, liver disease, and a variety of other complications related to alcohol abuse.

Patients without insurance represented 25% (n = 445) of the sample, with 29.1% (n = 383) of all pre-intervention recidivists being uninsured (χ^2 = 12.8, df = 1, p < .01). This rate dropped to 23.7% post-intervention with social work (χ^2 = 10.5, df = 1, p < .01). Patients transferred from other hospitals represented 15.4% (n = 272) of the sample, with 41.9% (n = 114) being uninsured. The variable Insurance was a reliable predictor for the variable Transfer (χ^2 = 46.8, df = 1, p < .01). This supports Ponto and Berg's (1992) assertion that public hospitals bear the brunt of medical costs accrued by the uninsured.

CASE EXAMPLES

Fred is a 43 year-old, sporadically employed white male with a long history of alcohol abuse. He resides at a local homeless shelter,

FIGURE 4. Presence of Alcohol Among ED Recidivists Pre- and Post-Intervention

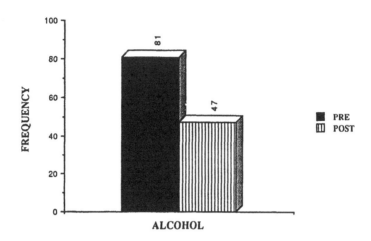

and receives Medicaid. His ED contacts began in early May when he was evaluated following an assault. He failed to return for follow-up removal of sutures; however, he was readmitted to the ED two weeks later reporting a second assault that left him unconscious for a short period of time. His sutures were removed and he was discharged. Within 24 hours he was returned to the ED after being found unconscious at the bottom of a 20-foot bridge. The EMS report assumed a fall. Fred was admitted to the hospital and spent two days in the ICU and four days on a general floor. The inpatient social worker evaluated him but he declined help with his alcohol problem. Three days post-discharge Fred was returned to the ED for seizures related to alcohol abuse. He was again treated and released. The following week he was brought in with seizures and impaired breathing. The social worker spent about an hour with him as his condition stabilized. He was frightened by his physical condition and expressed a desire for help with his drinking. Contact with a local substance abuse facility led to an admission for Fred that night. He was given a cab ride from the ED to the treatment facility. Fred was last seen in the ED approximately six weeks later when he voluntarily came in complaining of back pain from his earlier injury. He revealed that he had not been drinking, and his chart indicated that he had been following up with medical appointments. Fred expressed fear about returning to alcohol, and he was strongly reinforced by the ED staff for his sobriety and continued participation in his recovery program.

Susan is a 27 year-old white female with a lengthy history of repeated visits to this and other EDs starting in adolescence. She frequently presented with complaints of falling and back pain. She had several psychiatric hospitalizations and numerous psychiatric consults leading to diagnoses of borderline personality disorder in combination with either a disassociative disorder or a factitious disorder. At the time of this study, she had been seen in the ED three times over the previous four months with increasingly severe injuries sustained from a drug abusing significant other. On the fourth visit, the social worker found Susan responsive to discussing the destructive nature of the relationship. When she verbalized a willingness to accept help from the local domestic violence project, the worker immediately contacted them for assistance. They came to the ED and the patient was discharged to their residence. Susan was seen in follow-up three months later when she came to the ED complaining of a migraine headache. She was accompanied by staff from the domestic violence program, reported that she continued to live at their residence, and noted that she was employed for the first time in a number of years.

DISCUSSION

Interventions associated with the greatest decline in recidivism among patients with a non-medical diagnosis were those that required an active and anticipatory stance on the part of the social worker. As shown in Figure 2, the greatest decline in recidivism occurred in those categories where social work used a proactive intervention strategy as opposed to a more support-oriented intervention. This result is consistent with Moonilal's (1982) conclusion about the need for an active stance in ED social work. Acceptance of social work by medical personnel as a "team member" with full access to the patient is thus essential as restriction to formal evaluation compromises the social work contribution to ED patient care.

Social workers are especially trained to address the myriad of issues presented in the ED by recidivists and patients with non-medical complaints. Previous to social work's presence in the ED at UMMC non-medical complaints went largely unaddressed due to the nature of the setting and the absence of appropriate personnel to emergently address psychosocial aspects of the patient. This study has demonstrated that social work can reduce recidivism, improve quality of care, and contain the cost of uninsured recidivists presenting non-medical complaints who inappropriately use the ED of a high volume emergency medical department.

CONCLUSION

Social work in the Emergency Department can impact the recidivism rates of patients with non-medical complaints. However, the availability and knowledge of community resources (e.g., homeless shelters, detox centers, community mental health, women's crisis centers, etc.) is critical to the effectiveness of ED social work. With many community programs struggling to survive under the threat of budget cuts, EDs may become the kindest, yet most costly common ground for patients best served in their community. Triaging patients to specific community-based resources is cost-effective, and emphasizes the unique needs of each patient. Still, the question of ED social work follow-up post-discharge to community resources remains undocumented, and could be one avenue for expanding the role of ED social work in an effort to provide even more comprehensive and cost-effective care.

REFERENCES

Bennett, M.J. (1973). The social worker's role. *Hospitals, 47*(10), 111-118.
Boyack, V.J., & Bucknum, A.E. (1992). The quick response team: A pilot project. *Social Work in Health Care, 16*(2), 55-68.
Corr, J.M. (1992). Mind over matter. *Harvard Health Letter, 17*(6), 4-5.
Dove, H.G., Schneider, K.C., & Gitelson, D.A. (1985). Identifying patients who need social work services: An interdisciplinary analysis. *Social Work, 30,* 214-218.
Lindenberg, R.E. (1972). The need for crisis intervention in hospitals. *Hospitals, J.A.H.A., 46,* 52-55.
Moonilal, J.W. (1982). Trauma centers: A new dimension for hospital social work. *Social Work in Health Care, 7*(4), 15-25.

Ponto, J.M., & Berg, W. (1992). Social work services in the emergency department: A cost-benefit analysis of an extended coverage program. *Health and Social Work, 17*(1), 66-73.

Silverman, E. (1986). The social worker's role in shock-trauma units. *Social Work, 31*, 311-313.

Strinsky, C. (1970). Medical social worker. *Hospitals, J.A.H.A., 44*, 58-60.

Negative Experiences in Support Groups

Maeda J. Galinsky, PhD
Janice H. Schopler, PhD

SUMMARY. Although the benefits of support groups are well documented in the literature, little attention has been given to possible negative effects. A review of the literature related to support groups, negative experiences in groups, and social support, as well as personal accounts of members and practitioners, affirm the importance of considering the negative experiences in support groups. In addition, this material provides a base for the specification of potential problematic group conditions and negative outcomes and points to issues in obtaining information from respondents about negative factors. Findings from mailed questionnaires given to practitioners leading cancer support groups indicate the nature of the negative experiences in groups that these practitioners had led or heard about. Implications of these findings for prevention and intervention are discussed.

The benefits of support groups for people who share common stresses are widely publicized and seldom questioned. Both the professional literature and the popular media provide frequent reports of the relief, reassurance, practical information, guidance, and enhanced coping skills that members of support groups gain as they share their experiences. Because human service professionals recognize the positive outcomes that are associated with this mutual approach to helping, they are offering an increasing number of

Maeda J. Galinsky and Janice H. Schopler are affiliated with the School of Social Work, University of North Carolina at Chapel Hill, 223 E. Franklin Street, CB# 3550, Chapel Hill, NC 27599-3550.

[Haworth co-indexing entry note]: "Negative Experiences in Support Groups." Galinsky, Maeda J., and Janice H. Schopler. Co-published simultaneously in *Social Work in Health Care* (The Haworth Press, Inc.) Vol. 20, No. 1, 1994, pp. 77-95; and: *Social Work in Ambulatory Care: New Implications for Health and Social Services* (ed: Gary Rosenberg, and Andrew Weissman) The Haworth Press, Inc., 1994, pp. 77-95. Multiple copies of this article/chapter may be purchased from The Haworth Document Delivery Center [1-800-3-HAWORTH; 9:00 a.m. - 5:00 p.m. (EST)].

77

support group services to help people deal with common crises, life transitions, or chronic conditions. As the support group movement has gathered momentum, some systematic attention has been given to conceptualizing and evaluating support groups, but the possible negative effects of support group participation have received little attention.

There seems to be an assumption that outcomes for participants in support groups are uniformly positive, but that assumption is neither supported by research nor experience. This paper first addresses the importance of considering negative experiences in support groups and identifies the problems related to obtaining information about negative factors. Then, data from practitioners leading cancer support groups are presented and the implications for prevention and intervention are examined.

WHY FOCUS ON THE NEGATIVE?

Concern with the negative experiences in support groups is rooted in the commitment of social work and other human service professionals to promote individual and social well-being. There is ample evidence that support group members may gain substantial benefits from their participation and that support groups are a highly effective helping approach for many people. A review of the literature indicates, however, that the potential for negative outcomes exists. This conclusion is borne out by personal communications to the authors and exploratory research that demonstrates the problems and negative experiences that occur in these groups. Unfortunately, the negative impact of support groups is seldom reported or discussed.

Human service professionals have both an ethical and legal responsibility to do no harm, but support group leaders may be ill-prepared to prevent and deal with negative effects. Popular acclaim of the benefits of support groups coupled with the positive thrust of the professional and research literature creates a climate that discourages open discussion of negative dimensions. Practitioners are neither alerted to the negative aspects of support groups nor provided with any guidance about how to prevent or deal with problems and issues. The intent of this study is to promote a more balanced view of support group outcomes so that practitioners will be better prepared to maximize the benefits of support groups.

Support groups can be viewed as the center of a continuum overlapping with self-help groups (also referred to as mutual help groups) at one extreme and treatment groups at the other. Support groups are often facilitated by professional leaders and, sometimes, by volunteers. A primary focus in support groups is the development of reciprocal helping relationships among members so that the group can become both a supportive environment and a potential means for developing the capabilities of the members (Schopler & Galinsky, 1993).

Although there has been little attention to negative features of support groups, in this study negative support group outcomes include a range of outcomes from negative effects for members (e.g., member distress, decline in member functioning, disruption of positive member relations with individuals and organizations) to group problems and the ethical and legal concerns of practitioners. The negative effects for members are associated with negative experiences in the group. Negative experiences stem from problematic group processes which are unnecessarily stressful, and from processes related to group development which are inadequately addressed by the leaders (Galinsky & Schopler, 1981). It is important to note that some painful and conflictual group processes are expected in the course of group development and can enhance the experience of members with skillful facilitation by the leader.

Examination of several areas of the literature are particularly relevant to the study of negative factors. The practice literature related to groups provides evidence of negatives in a broad range of groups. The support group literature includes some limited discussion of negative features that have been specifically examined in support groups. The social science literature on social relationships addresses the conceptualization of negative interpersonal relationships and examines their impact on social networks.

The potential for negative experiences in therapy, personal growth, and disease management groups has been noted in both the theoretical and research literature related to group practice (Galinsky & Schopler, 1977; Lieberman, Yalom, & Miles, 1973; Roback, 1984; Schopler & Galinsky, 1981). The properties associated with these group experiences and their implications for professional responsibility and ethical behavior are recognized by group leaders in a range of helping professions (Lakin, 1988). Similar concerns have been raised about self-help groups (Chesler, 1990). For example, because leaders share influence with members in these groups, the leader has less control than in individual helping approaches and negative forces can arise because groups encourage both expressiveness and mutual helping. Further, group members are peers who typically have no professional training or accountability, yet they may feel pressure to participate. Thus, based on superficial knowledge, their own despair, or other personal motivations, they may make statements or give feedback that is misguided, unhelpful, and even harmful. While rarely examined in the support group literature, these same group properties are likely to characterize support groups. In fact, the value placed on shared experiences in support groups tends to give members more influence. This factor, coupled with the open-ended nature of many support groups, suggests that support groups may offer more opportunities for negative events but less awareness of their occurrence, since follow-up and evaluation are often complicated by members coming and going.

A review of the support group literature reveals that almost all accounts relate only to successful group experiences. Although some evaluations of support groups have been conducted, most studies measure only positive outcomes and tend to ignore negative effects. The exceptions include: Borkman's (1984) explication of the ways that personal networks can be unsupportive; Richman's (1989) study of hospice groups which finds that open communication can be threatening and that support group participation can increase stress and tension; and, Schopler and Galinsky's (1993) exploratory study of support groups as open systems.

Developments in the general study of social relationships over the past decade have drawn attention to negative as well as supportive aspects of informal social networks (Harris, 1992; Rook, 1992; Shumaker & Brownell, 1984). These studies have focused on the interactions of dyads in these networks. Exchanges are viewed as negative or problematic when they cause a person to experience some psychological distress and to have some reservations about the relationship (Rook, 1992). Some of the negative effects that have been noted for individuals in social interactions are pressures to conform, stresses related to reciprocal obligations, feeling overwhelmed and less adequate, learning inappropriate responses, embarrassment, and over-confidence (Shumaker & Brownell, 1984). These types of negative social interactions may be magnified in a support group.

This focus on the negative is not intended to exaggerate the prevalence or impact of interpersonal tensions and conflicts in social relationships nor to minimize the benefits that can be obtained from supportive social interactions. Rather, as Rook (1992) points out, a comprehensive understanding of both kinds of experiences is needed to design effective social interventions. To date, social network interventions have tended to address only the need to create supportive relationships. Information about negative as well as positive exchanges would make it possible to be responsive to the need to improve the quality of relationships and the need to disengage when stresses outweigh benefits.

There is growing evidence that, while helpful and harmful interactions can take place within the same relationship, they do not necessarily offset each other. Fiore, Becker, and Coppel (1983), studying caregivers of spouses with Alzheimer's disease, questioned the tendency to measure social support as a global, unidirectional construct ranging from no support to more support. Fiore and colleagues (1983) independently assessed three factors: the perceived helpfulness of different types of social network support; the upsetting effects of the absence of expected or desired support; and, the presence of negative input. They found that the extent of upsetting effects was a stronger predictor of depression than the helpfulness/upset ratio and both measures predicted depression better than ratings of helpfulness alone. In a related study, Schuster, Kessler, and Aseltine (1990) found negative interactions to be more predictive of emotional functioning than supportive interactions for married couples. Although there was some evidence that supportive interactions buffer the effects of distressing interactions, they suggest that the absence of negative interactions may be more important to mental health than the presence of support. Further, Gurley (1991) found, in an ethnographic study of women who were abused as children, that behaviors that support and obstruct recovery can co-exist in intimate relationships. Thus, to understand how help and harm may offset one another, she points out they must be conceptualized as independent dimensions.

Rook (1992) provides a comprehensive review of the research on negative interactions that occur in informal social networks. She also suggests that a critical threshold may exist for both supportive and negative interactions. The threshold effect refers to the point at which increasing levels of positive or negative reinforcement will have little impact. If this is the case, increasing either supportive or negative interactions alone will have little impact on an individual's well-being once the threshold is reached. Thus, threshold effects may confound comparisons of supportive and problematic exchanges.

The possibility of threshold effects is of particular concern in light of the fact that Rook (1984) and other researchers have found that almost all respondents in their studies report some supportive interactions but only a small proportion report negative interactions. Further, Rook notes that individuals who are very deficient in support may tend to be underrepresented because they are often difficult to locate or may be reluctant to participate. As noted in the studies reviewed above, however, when negative interactions are reported, they tend to have a greater impact than supportive exchanges on psychological functioning (Fiore et al., 1983; Schuster et al., 1990; Gurley, 1991). Rook suggests that the apparent disproportionate impact of negative exchanges may result from collecting data that included the critical threshold for negative exchanges but excluded the critical threshold for positive exchanges. Thus, understanding of the relative influence of negative and positive exchanges may be enhanced by the use of explicit tests for threshold effects. It is especially important to study the interactive effects of positive and negative interactions within dyads and small groups to gain a better understanding of what kinds of interventions can prevent or reduce negative exchanges and maximize positive effects.

The authors' personal experiences and conversations with support group members and group leaders in the course of their consultation, teaching, and research affirm that participation in support groups can contribute to personal well-being and be immensely gratifying. It is also clear that these groups can be upsetting and create problems for their members. Listening to a variety of support group members confide their negative experiences has been instructive. These former support group members have sought out the authors and volunteered information about their experiences following classroom and workshop presentations about support groups. They have talked about how overwhelming and depressing they found group sessions. They heard other members talk about their deteriorating conditions, learned about distressing encounters with the medical and legal system, and sensed the despair of others who were in similar situations. In some cases, they also were given bad advice. The people who shared their reactions did not return to their support groups and sought other sources of support. Although the authors talked only with a limited number of support group members, the intensity of the feelings expressed validates the need to gain a better understanding of negative aspects of support groups so that they can be prevented or addressed.

An earlier pilot study of 12 support group leaders (Schopler & Galinsky, 1993) suggests, however, that there may be barriers to obtaining information about negative effects. In this study, group leaders rarely noted issues and problems and, when they did, they tended to say that negatives can be addressed with skilled facilitation. Thus, the issue of how to identify and quantify negative experiences must be addressed to obtain comprehensive data about the type and frequency of their occurrence in support groups. Furthermore, although it would be highly desirable to collect information from members, issues related to client confidentiality and access to clients need to be resolved to make this possible.

Several conclusions can be drawn from the review of the literature related to negative group experiences, support groups, the detrimental aspects of social relationships and from the authors' consultations with support groups' leaders. First of all, negative experiences can result from any social interaction. Secondly, gaining information about negative aspects of social relationships can be difficult to obtain. Finally, although positive features of support groups have been emphasized, a balanced perspective that includes both the positive and negative dimensions of group experiences, is critical for designing group interventions that provide social support. With these conclusions in mind, a study was designed to obtain information about both positive and negative experiences in groups. The specific research questions addressed in this report are: (1) What problems and issues occur in support groups? and (2) What are the negative effects of support group participation?

METHODOLOGY

Data were collected from oncology social workers because support groups are a widely accepted intervention in the health field, and are frequently offered as a service to persons with cancer and their significant others (Berger, 1984; Cordoba, Shear, Fobair & Hall, 1984; Chesney, Rounds & Chesler, 1989; Galinsky, 1985; Patenaude, Levinger & Baker, 1986; Vugia, 1991). Access to a state-wide sample of support group leaders serving a defined population was an important consideration in selecting leaders of cancer support groups as the respondents for this pilot study. The study was limited to leader responses because lack of access to members and limited funding did not make it possible to expand the sample to support group members. All social workers who were members of the North Carolina Social Work Oncology Group (NCSWOG) were phoned to see if they were working with a group or if others in their agencies were facilitating such a group. Twenty support group leaders were located and all agreed to fill out a questionnaire giving information about their groups.

The questionnaire, mailed to respondents, was designed to elicit information on the characteristics of support groups as open systems, based on a model developed by Schopler and Galinsky (1993). Four conceptual dimensions are viewed as important: environmental conditions; participant characteristics; group conditions; and outcomes. Data were collected on all four dimensions through a structured questionnaire with fixed choice responses. This paper focuses on the outcome dimension and highlights negative effects for members, group problems, and ethical and legal concerns.

To obtain information about potentially negative group conditions, respondents were asked about problems and issues that they were informed had been cited in the literature or mentioned by groups' leaders. The categories of problems and issues listed in the questionnaire were compiled from a review of the literature related to group services and from the authors' consultations and workshops. Respondents were first asked if these problems and issues had occurred in their current support group and then asked if these problems and issues had occurred in other groups which they had heard about or which they had observed or led. The wording and sequence of questions were intended to normalize the occurrence of negative experiences in groups so that respondents would be more willing to share this type of information. The same procedure was used to gather data about negative effects for members. Respondents were also queried about their concerns about particular ethical and legal issues that had been noted in the literature or by practitioners. In addition, leaders were given a list of several interventions and were asked to indicate which approaches, if any, they had used to deal with problems and negative effects in their own groups.

Respondents indicated on the questionnaire their willingness to provide further information about support groups in a telephone interview. If they answered affirmatively, an appointment was made for a 15 to 30 minute telephone interview which focused on the negative factors that they had noted on their mailed questionnaires, as well as their suggestions for group leadership of support groups. Of the twenty persons who responded to the initial surveys, twelve agreed and were subsequently interviewed.

FINDINGS

A brief summary of some of the environmental conditions, participant characteristics, and group conditions gives a sense of the support groups in which the respondents played a leadership role. The primary sponsors of the 20 groups in the study were hospitals (12), hospices (5) and the American Cancer Society (3). All of the leaders had professional degrees; 14 of the respondents were social workers. Eighteen of the respondents worked with one or more co-leaders. Over half of the groups (11) were composed of both family members and patients; seven were for family members only; and, two were confined to patients. In 18 of the groups, both women and men were members. Fourteen of the groups were multiracial; the other six had only white members. All but one of 20 groups were open-ended. The goals rated as "very important" in these groups included emotional support (19 groups), guidance/advice

(18 groups), information (16 groups), problem-solving (12 groups), skill-building (6 groups) and individual change (4 groups). The groups in the sample used several approaches to goal achievement: 19 used open discussion; 14 considered specific topics; 9 had guest speakers; 5 became involved in advocacy activities; 4 used exercises/role plays; and, 4 used films and videos.

Table 1 provides data on the benefits that leaders noted for members of the support groups that they were currently leading. The benefits cited by leaders are ordered in terms of the frequency with which they were checked. As can be seen, respondents felt that the support groups they led provided many positive outcomes for their members. Each benefit was checked by at least 13 respondents, and five of these benefits (i.e., feel accepted, opportunity to hear different perspectives, emotional release, sense of being cared for, and normalization of experience) were checked by all or all but one respondent.

Table 2 gives a picture of group problems and issues cited by respondents for their current groups and for "other" groups, those they had observed, previously led, or heard about. Group leaders did indicate that there were problems and issues in their current groups.

TABLE 1. Group Leader Reports of Benefits in Their Current Cancer Support Groups (N = 20)

Benefits	No. of Leaders Reporting
Feel accepted	20
Opportunity to hear different perspectives	20
Sense of being cared for	19
Normalization of experience	19
Emotional release	19
Feeling of hope	17
Increased knowledge about cancer	16
Increased knowledge about resources	15
Feel relief and reassurance	15
Increased skill in dealing with cancer	15
Decreased fear and ambiguity	14
Friendship	14
Increased feeling of competence	13
Gratified by helping others	13

Foremost among these were factors leading to some degree of unpredictability and difference in the groups, namely irregular attendance, and members at different stages in dealing with cancer. In the same vein, failure to return/premature termination, and varied length of membership were the categories next most often checked. Problems in group interaction, i.e., lack of participation and disruptive members, were mentioned with a moderate degree of frequency.

Although there were some differences in the relative frequencies of problems and issues when group leaders were asked about their current groups and groups they had observed, previously led or heard about, the rankings given were fairly similar (rho = .68, p < .05). The top categories in both their current groups and other groups were irregular attendance and members at different stages in dealing with cancer. However, group-based problems, such as lack of participation, disruptive member(s), and unclear goals were giv-

TABLE 2. Group Leader Reports of Problems in Their Current Groups and Other Cancer Support Groups (N = 20)

Problems	No. of Leaders Reporting	
	Current Group	Other Groups[a]
Irregular Attendance	15	18
Members at different stages	15	15
Premature Termination	7	7
Varied length of membership	7	5
Lack of participation	6	14
Disruptive members	4	12
Unclear Goals	2	10
Other problems/issues	2	1
Overly dependent	1	7
Inappropriate Composition	1	5
Inappropriate Behavior	1	1
Interpersonal Conflicts	0	5
Confidentiality Violated	0	3
Fail to follow group norms/rules	0	3

[a]Other groups include groups that respondents had previously led, observed, or heard about

en higher rankings in other groups than in the current groups that the respondents were leading. Somewhat lower rankings in other groups were given to premature termination and varied length of membership.

Table 3 contains information about respondents' perception of negative effects for members in their current groups and in other groups. The data are organized, as for group issues and problems, with categories presented in order of the leaders' ranking for their current groups. Rankings of negative effects were very similar for current groups and for other groups (rho = .90, p < .01). Some negative outcomes were noted by one quarter to one half of respondents for current groups (i.e., find open communication threatening, experience sense of loss when member leaves, and feel overwhelmed); other negative effects were cited infrequently or not at all. Overall, negative effects were checked more frequently for

TABLE 3. Group Leader Reports of Negative Effects in Their Current and Other Cancer Support Groups (N = 20)

| | No. of Leaders Reporting | |
Negative Effects	Current Group	Other Groups[a]
Find open communication threatening	9	13
Sense of loss when member leaves	7	11
Feels overwhelmed	5	9
Becomes too dependent on group	4	7
Embarrassment	3	8
Sense of loss when group ends	3	7
Appears distressed	3	9
Learning inappropriate behavior	2	5
Obtaining incorrect information	1	5
Other negative effects	1	0
Feel pressure to conform	0	2
Stressed by group obligations	0	3
Becoming overconfident	0	1
Feeling excluded/different/scapegoated	0	2

[a]Other groups include groups that respondents had previously led, observed or heard about

other groups, and all categories were checked at least once by respondents for other groups. This difference in absolute numbers is to be expected since the pool from which respondents could draw was larger for the other category than for their single, current group experience.

Table 4 presents data on leader concerns about selected ethical or legal issues. As can be seen, respondents expressed some concerns about confidentiality, norms that encourage inappropriate behavior, and legal liability for destructive behavior stemming from group participation. When leaders were asked about the approaches that they used in their current support group for dealing with group problems and negative effects for members, almost all respondents indicated they provided direction (see Table 5). Group problem-solving and individual contact with members were also frequently employed. Structured exercises and activities were rarely used.

The telephone interview data from twelve group leaders provided an elaboration of the information given in the mailed question-naires. These leaders were very willing to share their observations and experiences and to offer suggestions for minimizing negative aspects. Several leaders spoke of the ways in which persons might be negatively affected by hearing the experiences of members with more advanced cases of cancer and by a premature breakdown of their systems of protective denial. Respondents stated that persons with cancer who are referred to support groups do not necessarily want to discuss feelings in a group and leaders suggested that some individuals should be allowed just to listen. Furthermore, as one respondent noted, "support groups aren't for everyone." Leaders spoke of their own frustration about irregular attendance patterns

TABLE 4. Group Leader Reports of Concerns They Have About Cancer Support Groups (N = 20)

Concerns	No. of Leaders Reporting
Questions about confidentiality	11
Norms that encourage inappropriate behavior	7
Concerned about legal liability for group-related destructive behavior	4

TABLE 5. <u>Group Leader Reports of Approaches Used to Deal with Group Problems and Negative Effects in Cancer Support Groups</u> (N = 20)

Approaches	No. of Leaders Reporting
Leader provides direction	18
Use group problem-solving	11
Individual contact with members	9
Structured exercise/activities	2

and of the emotional stress they face as oncology social workers. They noted that leaders need to keep some emotional distance to maintain a balanced perspective and pointed out that co-leadership can be helpful for leader support and for dealing with negative experiences. Some leaders stated that medical knowledge, or the accessibility of the group to a medical professional, was critical for answering questions and preventing misinformation. Respondents emphasized the importance of group work education, training, and experience for leadership of support groups.

DISCUSSION

Support groups are viewed in a positive light by the practitioners who lead them. They are seen as offering many benefits to their members. However, the picture of support groups is not completely positive. Problems and issues arise in the groups and there are negative effects for members. These negative aspects are a cause for consideration, although not necessarily for alarm. How to prevent negative aspects of group functioning when possible; how to deal with inevitable issues; and how to intervene in the group or with individual members when negative experiences occur are all critical questions for practice with support groups.

The data reported here are part of a pilot project and the findings are regarded as suggestive. The sample was drawn from organizations which had members in the North Carolina Social Work Oncology Group in the fall of 1991 and the spring of 1992, and generalizations apply solely to this population. Additional support group samples need to be studied to obtain a more representative overall sample and to understand similarities as well as differences in populations who use these types of services.

Practitioners only were asked about their observations; perceptions of other agency personnel, of group members and of their families and friends were not solicited, restricting the nature of the information collected. Although problems related to gaining access to members and limited funding prevented this line of inquiry, it is especially important to obtain data from group members. Only members can gauge the actual impact of group events and place them in the context of the total group experience. Furthermore, Lieberman and his colleagues (1973) found that participants were more likely to be aware of negative effects than were leaders. In addition, observations of meetings might be used to increase the validity of the data.

The nature of the problems and issues and negative effects for members reported are restricted partially by the fixed choice categories used in the questionnaire. These categories were developed from a review of the literature related to non-supportive social interactions, ethical concerns, and problems in group functioning, from prior interviews with practitioners and from the authors' knowledge of negative group functioning through research, consultation and teaching. Few respondents reported additional information about negatives and other means of expanding categories should be explored.

Leaders of support groups recognize that negatives do occur. Some of the problems and issues, such as irregular attendance and members at different stages of dealing with their condition, were noted previously for all types of open-ended groups (Galinsky & Schopler, 1987). To the extent that group issues and problems found in support groups are universal, education about group practice will be beneficial. However, it is also important to understand the uniqueness of support groups and to be prepared to deal with the special issues and problems they present. Leaders should recognize that persons who would not join other types of groups that provide assistance may join support groups because of their general popularity in our society or because of special crises they face.

Negative effects for members of the groups in our sample were not very frequent nor were they severe. They were numerous enough, however, to warrant attention. Casualties of the type studied by Lieberman et al. (1973), i.e., psychological distress and/or more maladaptive functioning that endured for at least eight months after the group experience, were not mentioned. This may be because these more extreme negative effects did not occur, because leaders did not have information about members after they left the group, or because leaders were not attuned to major negative effects in their own groups. Furthermore, cancer support groups are different from encounter or therapy groups and there may be fewer negative effects in support groups because of diminished pressure to reveal personal thoughts and feelings, fewer group confrontations and lowered expectations of personal transformation. However, because of the potential for negative effects, it is important to study further the negative impact for individuals who are members of support groups.

Respondents were trained leaders and were prepared to deal with problems and issues and with negative effects for members in their groups. They offered good ideas for how to intervene and gave clear evidence of the importance of appropriate training for group leadership. Their responses suggest that education about the leadership process and the potential for negative experiences is essential. Group facilitators need to be trained to understand factors that can impede group process as well as those conflictual elements that are a normal part of a group's development. An ability to assess the constructive or destructive potential of group issues and problems and an ability to deal with both positive and negative effects are important skills for group leaders. Thus, basic education about group work practice through formal classes and workshops is critical for all leaders, especially when staff and volunteers have not had formal training in practice with groups. Ongoing training and supervision are also required to maintain and develop leader sensitivity and skill in preventing and dealing with negative experiences. Further, manuals for practice with support groups, similar to that written by Cordoba, Shear, Fobair, and Hall (1984) for leadership of cancer support groups, need to be developed.

Unlike the experience of the authors in their initial study of support groups (Schopler & Galinsky, 1933), information on negative effects, group problems, and ethical and legal concerns was obtained in the present research. Practitioners reported a fair number of issues, problems and negative effects. There was a high, significant correlation between the rankings of issues and problems and negative effects for leaders' current groups and other groups, indicating a willingness of leaders to look at negative aspects in their own groups. In order to get this information, we constructed the questionnaires to "normalize" negative aspects, to make them an expected part of practice. We pointed to practice literature and to prior leader experience in the wording of the questions about negative aspects and we also asked for information about other groups, thus taking the complete focus off of the current group situation. Continued work on means of gathering reliable and valid data about negative aspects of support groups is required in order to build an effective practice base.

CONCLUSIONS

Guidelines for practice with support groups that recognize the possibilities of problems, issues, and negative effects in groups need to be more systematically developed and promoted. The literature review and pilot study presented in this paper are initial steps in the development of a practice theory for support groups that acknowledges negative aspects of group services and offers practice principles for prevention and intervention. There is a need to expand knowledge of negative experiences as one basis for developing these guidelines and providing education to professionals and volunteers. This type of leadership training is critical as the number of support groups proliferate and the need for group leadership increases.

AUTHOR NOTE

The authors express their thanks to Kristin Augustine, our graduate research assistant, for her support and contributions to this project and to the group leaders for their valuable information and their time.

This research was partially supported by a grant from the University Research Council at the University of North Carolina at Chapel Hill. An earlier version of this paper was presented at the 14th Annual Symposium of the Association for the Advancement of Social Work with Groups, Atlanta, GA, October, 1992.

REFERENCES

Berger, J. (1984). Crisis Intervention: A drop-in support group for cancer patients and their families. *Social Work in Health Care, 10*(2), 81-92.

Borkman, T. (1984). Mutual self-help groups: Strengthening the selectively un-supportive personal and community networks of their members. In A. Gardner & F. Riessman (Eds.), *The self-help revolution* (pp. 205-215). New York: Human Sciences Press.

Chesler, M.A. (1990). The "dangers" of self-help groups: Understanding and challenging professionals' views. In T.J. Powell (Ed.), *Working with self-help* (pp. 301-324). Silver Spring, MD: NASW Press.

Chesney, B., Rounds, K., & Chesler, M.A. (1989). Support for parents of children with cancer: The value of self-help groups. *Social Work with Groups, 12*(4), 119-139.

Cordoba, C., Shear, M.B., Fobair, P., & Hall, J. (1984). *Cancer support groups: Practice handbook.* Oakland, CA: American Cancer Society, California Division, Inc.

Fiore, J., Becker, J., & Coppel, D.B. (1983). Social network interactions: A buffer or a stress. *American Journal of Community Psychology, 11*(4), 423-439.

Galinsky, M.J. (1985). Groups for cancer patients and their families: Purposes and group conditions. In M. Sundel, P. Glasser, R. Sarri, & R. Vinter (Eds.), *Individual change through small groups* (pp. 519-532) (2nd ed.) New York: The Free Press.

Galinsky, M.J., & Schopler, J.H. (1987). Practitioners' views of assets and liabilities of open-ended groups. In J. Lassner, K. Powell, & E. Finnegan (Eds.), *Social group work: Competence and values in practice* (pp. 83-98). New York: The Haworth Press, Inc.

Galinsky, M.J., & Schopler, J.H. (1977). Warning: Groups can be dangerous. *Social Work, 22*, 88-91.

Gurley, D. (1991). The mixed roles of social support and social obstruction in recovery from child abuse. In D.D. Knudsen & J.L. Miller (Eds.), *Abused and battered: Social and legal responses to family violence* (pp. 88-99). New York: Walter de Gruyter, Inc.

Harris, T.O. (1992). Some reflections on the process of social support and nature of unsupportive behaviors. In H.O. Veiel & U. Baumann (Eds.), *The meaning and measurement of social support* (pp. 171-190). New York: Hemisphere Publishing Co.

Lakin, M. (1988). *Ethical issues in the psychotherapies.* New York: Oxford University Press.

Lieberman, M.A., Yalom, I.D., & Miles, M.B. (1973). *Encounter groups: First facts.* New York: Basic Books.

Patenaude, A.F., Levinger, L., & Baker, K. (1986, Fall). Group meetings for patients and spouses of bone marrow transplant patients. *Social Work in Health Care, 12*(1), 51-65.

Richman, J.M. (1989). Groupwork in a hospice setting. *Social Work with Groups, 12*(4), 171-184.

Roback, H.B. (1984). Conclusion: Critical issues in group approaches to disease management. In H.B. Roback (Ed.), *Helping patients and their families cope with medical problems* (pp. 527-543). San Francisco, CA: Jossey-Bass.

Rook, K.S. (1984). The negative side of social interaction. *Journal of Personality and Social Psychology, 46,* 1097-1108.

Rook, K.S. (1987). Reciprocity of social exchange and social satisfaction among older women. *Journal of Personality and Social Psychology, 52*(1), 145-154.

Rook, K.S. (1992). Detrimental aspects of social relationships: Taking stock of an emerging literature. In H.O. Veiel & U. Baumann (Eds.), *The meaning and measurement of social support* (pp. 157-169). New York: Hemisphere Publishing Co.

Schopler, J.H., & Galinsky, M.J. (1993). Support groups as open systems: A model for practice and research. *Health and Social Work, 18*(3), 195-207.

Schopler, J.H., & Galinsky, M.J. (1981). When groups go wrong. *Social Work, 26,* 424-429.

Schuster, T.L., Kessler, R.C., & Aseltine, R.H., Jr. (1990). Supportive interactions, negative interactions, and depressed mood. *American Journal of Community Psychology, 18*(3), 423-437.

Shumaker, S.A., & Brownell, A. (1984). Towards a theory of social support: Closing conceptual gaps. *Journal of Social Issues, 40*(4), 11-36.

Vugia, H.D. (1991). Support groups in oncology: Building hope through the human bond. *Journal of Psychosocial Oncology, 9*(3), 89-107.

Appendix

THE DORIS SIEGEL MEMORIAL FUND COMMITTEE

Honorary Chairmen

Dr. Thomas C. Chalmers
Dr. S. David Promrinse
Dr. John W. Rowe

Executive Secretary

Dr. Gary Rosenberg

Committee

Mrs. Susan S. Bailis
Mrs. Robert M. Benjamin
Dr. Barbara Berkman
Mr. Philip Bernstein
Dr. Susan Blumenfield
Dr. Lawrence Cuzzi
Mrs. Bess Dana
Dr. Kurt W. Deuschle
Dr. Sally Fiath Dorfman
Ms. Kathy Forrest
Dr. Richard Gorlin
Dr. Katherine Grimm
Mrs. Gail G. Grob
Mrs. Cecil Hailperin
Dr. Joseph M. Hassett
Dr. Karen Kaplan
Mrs. Robert A. Levinson

Dr. Jane Isaacs Lowe
Michael G. MacDonald, Esq.
Ms. Jane B. Mayer
Miss Janice Paneth
Mrs. Marjorie Pleshette
Dr. Helen Rehr
Dr. David Rose
Dr. Maurice V. Russell
Mrs. Beatrice P. Sachs
Mrs. Marvin Schur
Dr. Cecil Sheps
Dr. Harry Spiera
Mrs. Elinor Stevens
Miss Judith Trachtenberg
Mrs. Frank L. Weil
Mrs. Mary Wolf
Dr. Alma A. Young

Index

T - #0253 - 101024 - C0 - 212/152/6 [8] - CB - 9781560246978 - Gloss Lamination